# FREE VIDEO

## *Essential Test Tips* Video from Trivium Test Prep!

Thank you for purchasing from Trivium Test Prep!
We're honored to help you prepare for your exam.
To show our appreciation, we're offering a

### FREE *Essential Test Tips* Video

Our video includes 35 test preparation strategies that will make you successful
on your big exam. All we ask is that you email us your feedback and describe
your experience with our product. Amazing, awful, or just so-so:
we want to hear what you have to say!

---

To receive your **FREE** *Essential Test Tips* **Video**, please email us at
**5star@triviumtestprep.com.**

---

**Include "Free 5 Star" in the subject line and the following information in your email:**

1. The title of the product you purchased.
2. Your rating from 1 – 5 (with 5 being the best).
3. Your feedback about the product, including how our materials helped you meet
   your goals and ways in which we can improve our products.
4. Your full name and shipping address so we can send your
   **FREE** *Essential Test Tips* **Video**.

If you have any questions or concerns please feel free to contact us directly at:
**5star@triviumtestprep.com.**

Thank you!

– Trivium Test Prep Team

# PTCB Exam Study Guide 2021-2022:

Rapid Review with Practice
Questions for the Pharmacy Technician
Certification Board Test

Elissa Simon

# Table of Contents

# Introduction

Congratulations on your choice to become a Certified Pharmacy Technician! By purchasing this book, you've taken an important step toward succeeding in your career. The next step is to do well on the Pharmacy Technician Certification Exam, which will require you to demonstrate knowledge of the concepts and skills essential to working as a pharmacy technician. This book will walk you through these concepts and skills and provide you with important test strategies and tactics. Even if it's been years since you graduated from high school or cracked open a textbook, don't worry—this book contains everything you'll need to pass the exam.

## What is the Pharmacy Technician Certification Exam?

The Pharmacy Technician Certification Exam (PTCE) is administered by the Pharmacy Technician Certification Board (PTCB). The exam assesses the knowledge and abilities needed to perform pharmacy technician work. By passing the PTCE, pharmacy technicians are nationally accredited and receive the title of a Certified Pharmacy Technician, or CPhT.

## How Do I Qualify for the PTCE?

To schedule a test, you must first get authorization from the PTCB showing you have met all the pre-qualifications. You have two pathways to meet these requirements.

- Pathway 1: completion of a PTCB-recognized education or training program
- Pathway 2: a minimum of 500 hours work experience as a pharmacy technician

After you receive authorization and pay the $129 test fee, you can schedule a test online or by phone with Pearson-VUE Professional Testing Centers.

## What's on the PTCE?

The PTCE is a computer-generated multiple-choice exam that contains 90 questions. Of the ninety questions, eighty questions are scored and ten questions are unscored. You will have 1 hour and 50 minutes to complete the exam.

The content covered on the PTCE is broken down into four categories: medications, federal requirements, patient safety and quality assurance, and order entry and processing. The table below shows the topics covered within each category and their weight on the exam.

## What's on the PTCE?

| KNOWLEDGE DOMAIN | TOPICS COVERED | PERCENT OF EXAM |
|---|---|---|
| Medications | Generic names, brand names, and classifications of medications<br>Therapeutic equivalence<br>Common and life-threatening drug interactions and contraindications<br>Strengths/dose, dosage forms, routes of administration, special handling and administration instructions, and duration of drug therapy<br>Common and severe medication side effects, adverse effects, and allergies<br>Indications of medications and dietary supplements<br>Drug stability<br>Narrow therapeutic index (NTI) medications<br>Physical and chemical incompatibilities related to non-sterile compounding and reconstitution<br>Proper storage of medications | 40 |
| Federal Requirements | Federal requirements for handling and disposal of non-hazardous, hazardous, and pharmaceutical substances and waste<br>Federal requirements for controlled substance prescriptions and DEA controlled substance schedules<br>Federal requirements for controlled substances<br>Federal requirements for restricted drug programs and related medication processing<br>FDA recall requirements | 12.5 |
| Patient Safety and Quality Assurance | High-alert/risk medications and look-alike/sound-alike medications<br>Error prevention strategies<br>Issues that require pharmacist intervention<br>Event reporting procedures<br>Types of prescription errors<br>Hygiene and cleaning standards | 26.25 |
| Order Entry and Processing | Procedures to compound non-sterile products<br>Formulas, calculations, ratios, proportions, alligations, conversions, Sig codes, abbreviations, medical terminology, and symbols for days supply, quantity, dose, concentration, dilutions<br>Equipment/supplies required for drug administration<br>Lot numbers, expiration dates, and National Drug Code (NDC) numbers<br>Procedures for identifying and returning dispensable, non-dispensable, and expired medications and supplies | 21.25 |

## What Happens After the Exam?

Scores are scaled between 1000 and 1600, and a score of 1400 is required to pass the exam. When you finish the exam, you will receive an official result at the testing center. Your official result will appear in your PTCB account within three weeks. Within 6 weeks, you will be sent an official certificate and wallet card stating you are a certified pharmacy technician. To keep your certification current, you will be required to re-certify every 2 years.

# Online Resources

To help you fully prepare for your Pharmacy Technician Certification Exam, Trivium includes online resources with the purchase of this study guide.

## Practice Test

In addition to the practice test included in this book, we also offer an online exam. Since many exams today are computer based, getting to practice your test-taking skills on the computer is a great way to prepare.

## Flash Cards

A convenient supplement to this study guide, Trivium's flash cards enable you to review important terms easily on your computer or smartphone.

## Cheat Sheets

Review the core skills you need to master the exam with easy-to-read Cheat Sheets.

## From Stress to Success

Watch From Stress to Success, a brief but insightful YouTube video that offers the tips, tricks, and secrets experts use to score higher on the exam.

## Reviews

Leave a review, send us helpful feedback, or sign up for Trivium promotions—including free books!

Access these materials at:
www.triviumtestprep.com/ptcb-online-resources

# 1 Medications

## Pharmacology

**Pharmacology** is the study of the origin, uses, preparation, and effects of drugs on the body systems. **Pharmacodynamics** is the branch of pharmacology that involves how a drug affects the body. The majority of drugs act on the system in two ways:

- mimicking or suppressing normal physiological processes in the body

- inhibiting the growth of certain microbial or parasitic organisms

Drugs cannot change the fundamental physiological processes that occur in the body—they can only change the rate at which they occur. Drug action occurs when the drug binds to receptors on a protein molecule in the body to activate or block a physiological process.

- An **agonist** binds to receptors and stimulates activity. For example, nitroglycerin is an agonist that results in the activation of enzymes which dilate blood vessels. Endogenous agonists (e.g., serotonin, epinephrine) are the molecules produced by the body that naturally bind to receptor sites.

- An **antagonist** binds to a receptor to block activity. For example, ACE inhibitors block the angiotensin converting enzyme (ACE) which normally causes blood vessels to constrict. The result is dilation in the blood vessels.

- Some drugs are **partial agonists**, meaning they only partially activate receptors.

To determine how much of a medication is needed to effectively treat a disease or condition, a therapeutic window is calculated, which measures the dose required for the medication to be effective against the amount of it that would cause adverse side effects. For example, warfarin (Coumadin), which is used for blood clotting, has a very narrow therapeutic window; its use must be monitored, and the effective dose must be adjusted based on blood testing and other factors.

 **HELPFUL HINT**

Anticholinergic drugs block activity at acetylcholine receptors in the parasympathetic nervous system. They relax smooth muscles and are used to treat conditions like asthma, overactive bladder, and tremors. Some antipsychotics and SSRIs are also anticholinergic drugs.

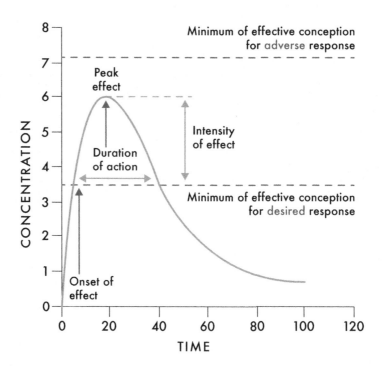

Figure 1.1. Therapeutic Window of Warfarin

Once the therapeutic window is determined, a duration of action is compiled, which is how long the drug will be effective. This usually relies on the peak concentration of the drug and is dependent upon the target plasma concentration—how much of the drug is present in a sample of plasma—required for the desired level of response.

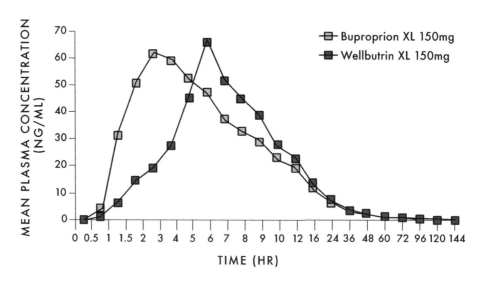

Figure 1.2. Bupropion's Duration of Action

## QUICK REVIEW QUESTION

1. Naloxone is an opioid antagonist. It reverses the effects of opioid overdose by

    A) acting as a central nervous system stimulant.

    B) removing opioids from the body.

    C) competitively binding to opioid receptors.

    D) reducing the production of endogenous opioids.

## Therapeutic Equivalence

The **brand name** of a drug is the name it is given by the pharmaceutical company that funded its research and development. This company holds the drug's patent for up to twenty years after its initial development, but when the patent expires, other pharmaceutical companies can produce the drug.

A **generic drug** is the therapeutic equivalent of the brand name of a drug. It must have the same active ingredient, strength, and dosage form as the brand-name drug, but the inactive ingredients do not need to be the same. Many generic drugs cost less to produce because generic manufacturers do not need to recoup the cost of research and development.

For the FDA to approve a generic drug, it must be **therapeutically equivalent** to the brand name, meaning it produces the same clinical effect and has the same safety profile. According to the FDA, therapeutic equivalent (generic) drugs must

- be as safe and effective as the brand name
- have the same active ingredients
- use the same route of administration
- be the same dosage
- meet the same manufacturing standards
- be bioequivalent (the same amount of usable drug reaches the body's circulation at the same rate)
- be correctly labeled

 **HELPFUL HINT**

Therapeutic equivalent drugs do NOT need to have the same appearance, packaging, preservatives, or flavor.

Generally, generic drugs can be substituted for prescribed brand-name medications (and vice versa) when the substitution will save the patient money. In fact, many insurers and state regulations require this substitution. *The Orange Book: Approved Drug Products with Therapeutic Equivalence Evaluations* identifies approved brand-name drug products along with evaluations of their therapeutic equivalents. *The Orange Book* is approved by the FDA, updated daily, and available online.

In some circumstances, generic drugs cannot be substituted for brand-name medications. Brand-name medications with a **narrow therapeutic index (NTI)** usually cannot be substituted with generic drugs. Small changes in dosages of NTI drugs can result in adverse events or therapeutic failure. Common NTI drugs include the following:

- carbamazepine
- cyclosporine
- digoxin
- levothyroxine
- lithium carbonate
- phenytoin
- warfarin

Providers and patients can also request either brand-name or generic drugs. Patient requests should always be honored; however, the patient should be advised that the brand-name drug may be more expensive or not covered by insurance.

A provider may use "**dispense as written**" **(DAW)** codes to indicate when a brand-name or generic drug is required. There are ten codes that can be used, but most insurance companies only recognize a few of them and strictly limit their use.

 **HELPFUL HINT**

If a prescription says "dispense as written" or "DAW," the pharmacy tech must dispense the exact medication as it is written on the prescription.

- DAW 0: No product selection is indicated. This code is used when it is acceptable to substitute the generic version of the drug.
- DAW 1: Substitutions are not allowed by the prescriber. This code is used when the doctor deems the brand medication to be medically necessary.
- DAW 2: The patient is requesting the brand-name version of the drug; this code is used when the patient will not take the generic, but the doctor does not deem the brand medically necessary.
- DAW 3: The pharmacist has selected the brand name although substitution is allowed.
- DAW 4: The generic version of the drug is not in stock; substitution is allowed.
- DAW 5: The brand-name version of the drug has been dispensed at the generic price; substitution is allowed.
- DAW 6: This is the override code.
- DAW 7: The brand-name drug is mandated by law; substitution is not allowed.
- DAW 8: The generic version of the drug is not available; substitution is allowed.
- DAW 9: other

2. A generic drug must have all the same characteristics as a brand-name drug EXCEPT its

   A) active ingredient.

   B) color.

   C) dosage.

   D) strength.

 **HELPFUL HINT**

Pharmacy technicians are not authorized to make therapeutic substitutions.

## Drug Classes

A **drug class** is a group of related medications that have the same mechanism of action or are used to treat the same condition. Drugs within a single drug class usually have the same suffix, although the suffixes of older drugs may differ because grouping generic drugs by suffix is a relatively new concept.

**Therapeutic substitution** is the substitution of a prescribed drug with another medication that produces the same therapeutic effect (usually from the same class). Often this substitution is done when a brand-name medication has no generic version, but a different generic drug is available in the same class. Pharmacists may offer therapeutic substitutes in some states, but prescriber approval is always required.

### TABLE 1.1. Drug Classes

| DRUG CLASS | COMMONLY USED SUFFIX | PURPOSE | EXAMPLE(S) GENERIC NAME (BRAND NAME) |
|---|---|---|---|
| alpha-adrenergic blockers | –azosin | relax the veins and arteries so blood can easily pass through; antihypertensives | terazosin |
| angiotensin II receptor blockers (A2RBs) | –artan | block angiotensin II enzymes from specific receptor sites; help prohibit vasoconstriction | candesartan |
| angiotensin converting enzyme (ACE) inhibitors | –pril | block the conversion of angiotensin I to angiotensin II; may reduce the chance of increased vasoconstriction or blood pressure | enalapril |
| antibiotics | –cillin –cycline –floxacin –mycin | inhibit growth of or kill bacteria | penicillin amoxicillin ciprofloxacin moxifloxacin vancomycin |
| anticoagulants (blood thinners) | N/A | prevent blood clots | rivaroxaban (Xarelto) warfarin (Coumadin) |

*continued on next page*

## TABLE 1.1. Drug Classes (continued)

| DRUG CLASS | COMMONLY USED SUFFIX | PURPOSE | EXAMPLE(S) GENERIC NAME (BRAND NAME) |
|---|---|---|---|
| anticonvulsants | N/A | prevent seizures | carbamazepine (Tegretol) topiramate (Topamax) |
| antidepressants | N/A | treat depression and mood disorders | fluoxetine (Prozac) sertraline (Zoloft) bupropion (Wellbutrin, Zyban) |
| antihistamines | N/A | treat allergies | diphenhydramine (Benadryl) |
| antipsychotics | N/A | manage psychosis | aripiprazole (Abilify) lithium carbonate |
| antivirals | –vir | inhibit growth of or kill viruses | docosanol (Abreva) oseltamivir (Tamiflu) |
| barbiturates | –barbital | depress the central nervous system | amobarbital (Amytal Sodium) butabarbital (Butisol) phenobarbital (Nembutal) |
| benzodiazepines | –pam | reduce anxiety and relax muscles | alprazolam (Xanax) clonazepam (Klonopin) lorazepam (Ativan) diazepam (Valium) |
| beta blockers (B1s) or beta-adrenergic blocking agents | –olol | reduce blood pressure and improve blood flow | acebutolol (Sectral) atenolol (Tenormin) metoprolol (Lopressor) propranolol (Inderal) |
| calcium channel blockers | –pine | relax and widen blood vessels | amlodipine (Norvasc) felodipine (Plendil) diltiazem (Cardizem) nifedipine (Procardia) |
| corticosteroids | –olone –sone | reduce inflammation | dexamethasone (Decadron) prednisone (Sterapred) |
| potassium-sparing diuretics | –actone | increase the flow of urine and enhance the loss of sodium | spironolactone |

| DRUG CLASS | COMMONLY USED SUFFIX | PURPOSE | EXAMPLE(S) GENERIC NAME (BRAND NAME) |
|---|---|---|---|
| loop diuretics | –emide | increase the flow of urine and enhance the loss of sodium | furosemide |
| histamine type-2 receptor antagonists (H2 blockers) | –tidine | reduce stomach acid | famotidine (PEPCID) ranitidine (Zantac) |
| HMG-CoA reductase inhibitors | –statin | inhibit cholesterol production | rosuvastatin (Crestor) |
| hypnotics | N/A | reduce anxiety and induce sleep | eszopiclone (Lunesta) zolpidem (Ambien) |
| immunosuppressants | N/A | suppress the immune system | adalimumab (Humira) methotrexate (Trexall) |
| local anesthetics | –caine | block sensation in a small area | lidocaine (Xylocaine, Lidoderm) benzocaine |
| neuromuscular blockers | –nium | paralyze skeletal muscles | pancuronium (Pavulon) rocuronium (Zemuron) |
| nonsteroidal anti-inflammatory drugs (NSAIDs) | N/A | reduce pain and inflammation | ibuprofen (Motrin, Advil) naproxen (Aleve, Naprosyn) |
| opioid pain relievers | –codone | block pain signals in brain | oxycodone (Percocet, OxyContin) morphine (Astramorph, Duramorph) |
| proton pump inhibitors | –razole | reduce stomach acid | esomeprazole (Nexium) lansoprazole (Prevacid) omeprazole (Prilosec) |

## QUICK REVIEW QUESTION

3. Drugs in a drug class must have the following traits in common EXCEPT

   A) the same targeted mechanism.

   B) a similar mode of action.

   C) the same active ingredient.

   D) similar structures.

# Medication Side Effects and Adverse Reactions

**Adverse drug reaction** is a broad term used to describe unwanted, uncomfortable, or dangerous effects caused by a specific medication. Most adverse drug reactions are dose related, but they can also be allergic or idiosyncratic (unexpected responses that are neither dose related nor allergic). Adverse drug reactions are one of the leading causes of morbidity and mortality in health care. They can be classified by severity as follows:

- mild (e.g., drowsiness)

- moderate (e.g., hypertension)

- severe (e.g., abnormal heart rhythm)

- lethal (e.g., liver failure)

**Allergic reactions** may cause itching, rash, airway edema with difficulty breathing, or a drop in blood pressure. Severe allergic reactions can cause anaphylaxis, which is a life-threatening condition requiring emergent care. An idiosyncratic reaction can cause almost any sign or symptom, and they usually cannot be predicted.

Adverse drug reactions are classified into six types.

**HELPFUL HINT**

A patient may continue taking a medication even if it has negative side effects. Some adverse reactions (e.g., dry mouth, diarrhea) subside with time, and sometimes the benefits of the drug outweigh the uncomfortable side effects. The patient should always check with the provider before discontinuing a medication.

**TABLE 1.2. Types of Adverse Drug Reactions**

| TYPE | DESCRIPTION | EXAMPLE |
|---|---|---|
| A augmented | predictable reactions arising from the pharmacological effects of the drug; dependent on dose | diarrhea due to antibiotics; hypoglycemia due to insulin |
| B bizarre | unpredictable reactions; independent of dose | hypersensitivity (anaphylaxis) due to penicillin |
| C chronic | reactions caused by the cumulative dose (the dose taken over a long period of time) | osteoporosis with oral steroids |
| D delayed | reactions that occur after the drug is no longer being taken | teratogenic effects with anticonvulsants |
| E end of use | reactions caused by withdrawal from a drug | withdrawal syndrome with benzodiazepines |
| F failure | unexpected failure of the drug to work; often caused by dose or drug interactions | resistance to antimicrobials |

4. Rifampin is an antibiotic used to treat tuberculosis. When taken with oral contraceptives, it can reduce estrogen levels and decrease the effectiveness of the contraceptive. This adverse reaction would be classified as

   A) A—augmented

   B) B—bizarre

   C) E—end of use

   D) F—failure

## Drug Interactions

Medications may interact with other medications or health conditions. These **drug interactions** can increase or decrease the action of the drug, which changes the therapeutic effects of the medication. There are three main types of drug interactions: drug-drug, drug-disease, and drug-nutrient.

In a **drug-drug interaction**, a person takes multiple medications. The drugs may be duplicates, meaning they have a similar therapeutic effect. This type of interaction can result in toxicity or increased effect. Combining drugs with opposite effects may reduce the effectiveness of one or both medications.

**Drug-disease interaction** occurs when a medication taken for one disease causes or exacerbates a different disease. For example, calcium channel blockers (to treat hypertension) must be used cautiously in patients with chronic kidney disease because they can impair kidney function.

Finally, drugs may interact with other consumable substances, including foods, alcohol, and nutritional supplements. These interactions are grouped together as **drug-nutrient interactions**. For example, alcohol and grapefruit juice both change the absorption and effectiveness of antibiotics.

## QUICK REVIEW QUESTION

5. Which of the following is an example of a drug-drug interaction?

   A) Taking omeprazole with clopidogrel may decrease the effectiveness of clopidogrel.

   B) Ibuprofen may cause or exacerbate gastrointestinal bleeding.

   C) Drinking grapefruit juice with simvastatin reduces the concentration of simvastatin in the blood.

   D) Antidepressants may cause suicidal thoughts or behaviors in children.

## Auxiliary Labels

**Auxiliary labels** are attached to the medication bottle to provide guidance to the patient on how medications should be taken or stored. These labels are not meant to replace counseling from the pharmacist. Instead, they should reinforce

**HELPFUL HINT**

Drug-drug interactions are common when patients take medications that contain multiple drugs. For example, a patient taking Norco and OTC Nyquil might not realize that both medications contain acetaminophen.

**HELPFUL HINT**

Monoamine oxidase inhibitors (MAOIs) are a class of antidepressants that are effective in treating mood disorders but are rarely used due to their potential for drug-drug interactions. Most drugs that affect serotonin, norepinephrine, or dopamine levels are contraindicated for patients taking MAOIs.

instructions given by the pharmacist, included in patient handouts, or written on the product label. Auxiliary labels usually address one of the following concerns:

- administration (e.g., for topical use; take with food)
- interactions (e.g., do not take with grapefruit)
- storage requirements (e.g., keep in refrigerator)

The use of auxiliary labels is not nationally regulated, but the US Pharmacopeial Convention (UPC) has guidelines for pharmacies to follow. Some commonly used auxiliary labels are included in the table below, but many others exist (and may appear on the exam).

## TABLE 1.3. Common Auxiliary Labels

| LABEL | DRUG EXAMPLES |
|---|---|
| Chew tablets before swallowing. | methylphenidate (chewable tablets) <br> Vyvanse (chewable tablets) |
| Do not drink alcoholic beverages when taking this medication. | metronidazole <br> CNS depressants <br> insulin <br> antidiabetics |
| Do not eat grapefruit or drink grapefruit juice while taking this medication. | statins <br> calcium channel blockers |
| Do not take dairy products, antacids, or iron preparations within one hour of taking this medication. | alendronate <br> tetracyclines <br> fluoroquinolones |
| Do not take this drug if you become pregnant. | ACE inhibitors <br> ARBs <br> statins <br> warfarin <br> NSAIDs <br> carbamazepine |
| May cause drowsiness/dizziness. | opioids <br> benzodiazepines <br> *Note: usually excludes drugs whose main effect is drowsiness* |
| Medication should be taken with plenty of water. | sulfonamide antibiotics <br> Bactrim |
| Avoid prolonged exposure to sunlight. | sulfonamide antibiotics <br> metronidazole <br> tetracyclines |
| Swallow whole; do not crush/chew. | all extended-release (ER) tablets and capsules <br> benzonatate |

| LABEL | DRUG EXAMPLES |
| --- | --- |
| Take medication on empty stomach. | macrolide antibiotics<br>Levothyroxine<br>sildenafil<br>tadalafil |
| Take medication with food. | NSAIDs<br>metformin<br>carvedilol<br>lovastatin |

## QUICK REVIEW QUESTION

6. The auxiliary label, "Take medication with food," would be attached to which of the following medications?

    A) sildenafil

    B) lorazepam

    C) metformin

    D) carbamazepine

## Drug Administration

One of the specific factors that influences a drug's bioavailability and how it distributes through the system is its **route of administration**. Pharmacy technicians should be familiar with common routes of administration and their abbreviations so that the correct drug can be dispensed:

- buccal (BUC): in the cheek
- inhalational (INH): through the mouth
- intramuscular (IM): into the muscle
- intranasal (NAS): through the nose
- intravenous (IV): into the vein
- oral (PO): by mouth
- rectal (PR): into the rectum
- subcutaneous (subcut): under the skin
- sublingual (SL): under the tongue
- transdermal (TOP): through the skin
- vaginal (PV): into the vagina

CONTINUE

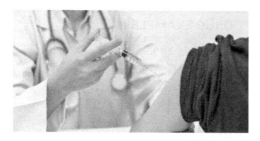

Intramuscular Injection

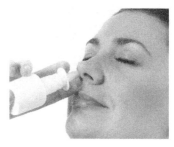

Intranasal Delivery

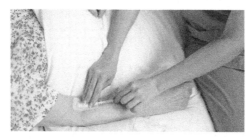

Intravenous Delivery

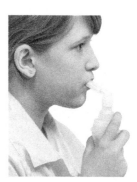

Inhalation

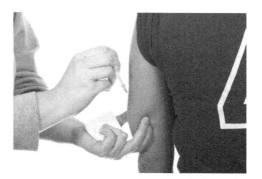

Subcutaneous Injection

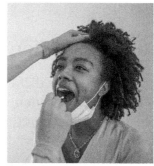

Buccal Delivery

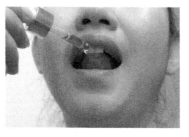

Sublingual Delivery

Figure 1.3. Routes of Administration

---

## QUICK REVIEW QUESTION

7. A patient has a prescription for nitroglycerin 0.4 mg SL. How should the patient be directed to take this medication?

   A) under the tongue

   B) in the cheek

   C) swallowed without chewing

   D) injected into the muscle

---

## The Cardiovascular System

The **cardiovascular system** circulates **blood**, which carries nutrients, waste, hormones, and other important substances dissolved or suspended in liquid plasma. Two of the most important components of blood are **white blood cells**, which fight infections, and **red blood cells**, which transport oxygen.

Blood is circulated by the heart, which is a muscular organ. The human heart has four chambers: the right and left atria and the right and left ventricles, as shown in Figure 1.4. Each chamber is isolated by valves that prevent the backflow of blood once it has passed through.

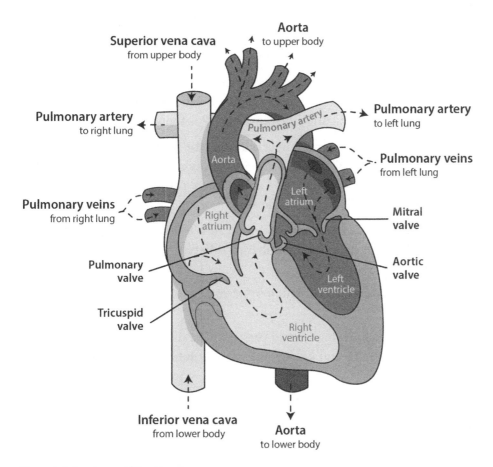

*Figure 1.4. Anatomy of the Heart*

Blood leaves the heart and travels throughout the body in **blood vessels**, which decrease in diameter as they move away from the heart and toward the tissues and organs. Blood exits the heart through **arteries**, which become **arterioles** and then **capillaries**, the smallest branch of the circulatory system in which gas exchange from blood to tissues occurs. Deoxygenated blood travels back to the heart through **veins**.

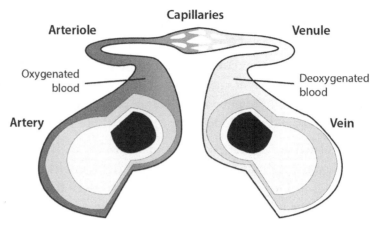

Figure 1.5. Blood Vessels

 **DID YOU KNOW?**

Many cardiac medications work by relaxing blood vessels (to decrease blood pressure) or constricting blood vessels (to increase blood pressure).

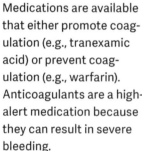 **HELPFUL HINT**

Medications are available that either promote coagulation (e.g., tranexamic acid) or prevent coagulation (e.g., warfarin). Anticoagulants are a high-alert medication because they can result in severe bleeding.

**HELPFUL HINT**

Some types of cholesterol worsen atherosclerosis. Statins (like Crestor and Zocor) lower cholesterol levels and reduce the risk of heart disease.

**Blood pressure (BP)** is the pressure exerted by blood on vessel walls. It is expressed as two numbers. The higher number is the **systolic BP**, which is found when the heart is contracting. The **diastolic BP** is found when the heart relaxes.

**Coagulation** is the formation of a **blood clot** (thrombus) to stop bleeding. Clots begin when specialized cells called **platelets** clump together to block blood flow. The activation of platelets is followed by a complex cascade of reactions involving proteins called **clotting factors**.

**Heart disease** is the most common cause of death in the United States. This umbrella term includes a number of different pathologies that cause the heart to weaken or stop:

- **Atherosclerosis**: hardening or narrowing of the arteries due to plaque deposits

- **Hypertension** (high blood pressure) is a risk factor for heart disease, stroke, and kidney disease. (**Hypotension** is decreased blood pressure.)

- **Myocardial infarction** (heart attack) is the death of heart tissue, typically caused by lack of blood flow to heart muscles due to a thrombus that blocks blood vessels.

- **Angina** is a small or temporary blockage in the heart's blood vessels that does not lead to tissue death.

- **Heart failure** occurs when either one or both ventricles in the heart cannot efficiently pump blood. It is typically due to another disease or illness, most commonly atherosclerosis.

- **Dysrhythmia** is an abnormal heart rhythm.

## TABLE 1.4. Cardiovascular Medications

| MEDICATION | COMMON BRAND NAMES | ADVERSE REACTIONS AND INTERACTIONS |
|---|---|---|
| **ACE INHIBITORS: *HYPERTENSION, HEART FAILURE*** | | |
| **lisinopril** | **Prinivil, Zestril** | **BBW:** fetal toxicity<br>**ADR:** cough, hypotension, dizziness<br>**Interactions:** other medications that lower BP |
| benazepril | Lotensin | |
| enalapril | Epaned, Vasotec | |
| ramipril | Altace | |
| **ANTICOAGULANTS: *THROMBUS PREVENTION*** | | |
| clopidogrel | Plavix | **BBW:** bleeding, abrupt discontinuation<br>**ADR:** bleeding<br>**Interactions:** omeprazole/esomeprazole (clopidogrel), NSAIDs<br>**Pregnancy:** Category X (warfarin, rivaroxaban) |
| warfarin | Coumadin; Jantoven | |
| apixaban | Eliquis | |
| rivaroxaban | Xarelto | |
| aspirin | Bayer | |
| **ANGIOTENSIN II RECEPTOR BLOCKERS (A2RBS): *HYPERTENSION, HEART FAILURE*** | | |
| losartan | Cozaar | **BBW:** fetal toxicity<br>**ADR:** dizziness, headache, fatigue<br>**Interactions:** potassium supplements, other drugs that lower BP<br>**Pregnancy:** Category D |
| losartan and hydrochlorothiazide | Hyzaar | |
| valsartan | Diovan | |
| valsartan and hydrochlorothiazide | N/A | |
| **BETA BLOCKERS: *HYPERTENSION, ANGINA, MIGRAINE, ANAPHYLAXIS*** | | |
| **metoprolol** | **Toprol-XL, Lopressor** | **BBW:** abrupt discontinuation<br>**ADR:** dizziness, fatigue, weight gain<br>**Interactions:** other drugs that lower BP |
| carvedilol | Coreg | |
| atenolol | Tenormin | |
| propranolol | Inderal, Hemangeol | |
| nebivolol | Bystolic | |
| timolol | none | |
| **CALCIUM CHANNEL BLOCKERS: *HYPERTENSION, ANGINA, DYSRHYTHMIAS*** | | |
| **amlodipine** | **Amvaz, Norvasc** | **ADR:** headache, edema, tiredness, dizziness<br>**Interactions:** other drugs that lower BP, grapefruit (nifedipine) |
| diltiazem | Cardizem | |
| nifedipine | Procardia | |
| verapamil | Calan, Verelan | |
| amlodipine and benazepril | Lotrel | |

*continued on next page*

## TABLE 1.4. Cardiovascular Medications (continued)

| MEDICATION | COMMON BRAND NAMES | ADVERSE REACTIONS AND INTERACTIONS |
|---|---|---|
| **HMG-COA REDUCTASE INHIBITORS (STATINS):** *HIGH CHOLESTEROL* | | |
| atorvastatin | Lipitor | **ADR:** muscle/joint pain<br>**Interactions:** grapefruit/grapefruit juice, some antibiotics (e.g., cyclosporine, clarithromycin), some antifungals (e.g., itraconazole)<br>**Pregnancy:** Category X |
| simvastatin | FloLipid, Zocor | |
| pravastatin | Pravachol | |
| rosuvastatin | Crestor | |
| lovastatin | Altoprev | |
| **OTHER ANTILIPEMICS:** *HIGH CHOLESTEROL* | | |
| fenofibrate | Tricor | **ADR:** abdominal/back pain, muscle/joint pain, headache, nausea, diarrhea<br>**Interactions:** grapefruit juice, anticoagulants, other drugs that lower cholesterol, cyclosporine (ezetimibe)<br>**Contraindications:** liver or gallbladder disease |
| gemfibrozil | Lopid | |
| ezetimibe | Zetia | |
| omega-3-acid ethyl esters (fish oil) | none | **ADR:** indigestion<br>**Interactions:** anticoagulants<br>**Contraindications:** fish or shellfish allergy |
| **VASODILATORS:** *ANGINA, HYPERTENSION* | | |
| hydralazine | Apresoline, Dralzine | **ADR:** headache, nausea/vomiting/diarrhea<br>**Interactions:** MAO inhibitors, other drugs that lower BP |
| isosorbide | none | **ADR:** dizziness, lightheadedness<br>**Interactions:** other drugs that lower BP, sildenafil, alcohol |
| nitroglycerin | none | |
| **MISCELLANEOUS** | | |
| digoxin<br>*dysrhythmias, heart failure* | Digitek, Digox, Lanoxin | **ADR:** nausea, diarrhea, headache, dizziness<br>**Interactions:** macrolide antibiotics, azole antifungals, other antidysrhythmic drugs |
| amiodarone<br>*dysrhythmias* | Nexterone, Pacerone | **BBW:** pulmonary toxicity<br>**ADR:** nausea, vomiting, dizziness, vision problems<br>**Interactions:** grapefruit juice |
| **BBW:** black box warning<br>**ADR:** adverse drug reactions | | |

 **HELPFUL HINT**

Aspirin is an NSAID that also slows platelet aggregation, which prevents clotting. It is often prescribed to prevent thrombus formation (e.g., myocardial infarction, stroke), but can also be taken for pain, fever, or inflammation.

## QUICK REVIEW QUESTIONS

**8.** Drugs with the suffix *–pril* are

   **A)** calcium channel blockers.

   **B)** beta blockers.

   **C)** fibric acid.

   **D)** ACE inhibitors.

**9.** Vasodilators lower blood pressure by

   **A)** reducing cholesterol levels.

   **B)** preventing coagulation.

   **C)** relaxing blood vessels.

   **D)** resetting the heart's rhythm.

**10.** A pharmacy technician should alert the pharmacist to counsel a patient who has presented prescriptions for both

   **A)** clopidogrel and furosemide.

   **B)** nitroglycerin and tadalafil.

   **C)** atorvastatin and benzonatate.

   **D)** lisinopril and amoxicillin.

## The Respiratory System

The **respiratory system** is responsible for the exchange of gases between the human body and the environment. Oxygen is brought into the body for use in glucose metabolism, and the carbon dioxide created by glucose metabolism is expelled.

Humans primarily take in air through the nose but can also do so through the mouth. Air travels down the **trachea**, **bronchi**, and **bronchioles** into the lungs. The **lungs** contain millions of small **alveoli** where oxygen and carbon dioxide are exchanged between the blood and the air.

> 💡 **HELPFUL HINT**
>
> A bronchospasm is a sudden constriction of the bronchioles that restricts airflow and is most commonly caused by asthma or COPD. It is treated with inhaled albuterol, which reopens the airway.

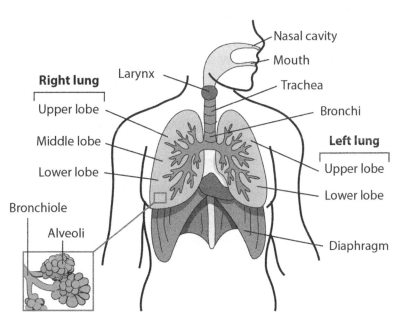

Figure 1.6. The Respiratory System

Respiratory disorders can be caused by infection or by pathophysiological processes that damage respiratory tract tissues.

- **Chronic obstructive pulmonary disease (COPD)** is a progressive restriction of airflow caused by constriction of airways and the destruction of lung tissue.

- **Asthma** is a chronic condition in which the airways narrow, swell, and produce excess mucus.

- Common **respiratory infections** include colds, influenza, and pneumonia. Children are at high risk for some more serious respiratory infections, including pertussis, croup, and bronchiolitis.

Many of the drugs used to treat respiratory problems can be purchased over the counter in both adult and child formulations.

- **Expectorants,** such as guaifenesin (Mucinex), help loosen up and thin mucus to make coughs more productive.

- **Antitussives** relieve coughing. Dextromethorphan is a common OTC antitussive.

- **Decongestants** help to relieve stuffy noses. Phenylephrine is the most common drug used in OTC decongestant medicines, although pseudoephedrine (Sudafed, Claritin-D, Allegra-D) is more effective. **Pseudoephedrine** purchases are highly regulated because they can be used to manufacture methamphetamine. (See chapter 2 for more on pseudoephedrine regulations.)

## TABLE 1.5. Respiratory Medications

| MEDICATION | COMMON BRAND NAMES | ADVERSE REACTIONS AND INTERACTIONS |
|---|---|---|
| **BRONCHODILATORS: *ASTHMA, COPD*** | | |
| albuterol | Ventolin HFA, Proventil HFA, Combivent Respimat, DuoNeb, ProAir HFA | **ADR:** headache, fast heart rate, dizziness, sore throat, nasal congestion<br>**Interactions:** beta blockers, digoxin, MAOI, tricyclic antidepressants |
| montelukast | Singulair | **BBW:** neuropsychiatric symptoms<br>**ADR:** respiratory infection, fever, headache, sore throat, cough |
| tiotropium | Spiriva | **ADR:** sore throat, cough, dry mouth, headache, visual disturbances<br>**Interactions:** other anticholinergics |
| ipratropium and albuterol | Combivent Respimat | **ADR:** upper respiratory infection, sore throat, cough, headache<br>**Interactions:** beta blockers, digoxin, MAOI, tricyclic antidepressants, other anticholinergics |

| MEDICATION | COMMON BRAND NAMES | ADVERSE REACTIONS AND INTERACTIONS |
|---|---|---|
| **BRONCHODILATORS AND CORTICOSTEROIDS: *ASTHMA, COPD*** | | |
| fluticasone and salmeterol | Advair Diskus/HFA, AirDuo RespiClick | **BBW:** worsening asthma symptoms (formoterol) **ADR:** respiratory infection, sore throat, oral candidiasis, cough, headache, nausea, vomiting **Interactions:** beta blockers, diuretics, MAOI |
| budesonide and formoterol | Symbicort | |
| **MISCELLANEOUS** | | |
| benzonatate *cough* | Tessalon | **ADR:** sedation, headache, congestion, "chilly" sensation in chest **Counseling:** Swallow capsule whole. |
| **BBW:** black box warning **ADR:** adverse drug reactions | | |

## QUICK REVIEW QUESTIONS

11. Which of the following medications may be prescribed for asthma?

   **A)** montelukast

   **B)** carvedilol

   **C)** doxycycline

   **D)** zolpidem

12. Which auxiliary label should be affixed to a prescription bottle of benzonatate?

   **A)** Do not take this drug if you become pregnant.

   **B)** Do not eat grapefruit or drink grapefruit juice while taking this medication.

   **C)** Keep refrigerated.

   **D)** Do not crush or chew; swallow whole.

## The Nervous System

The **nervous system** processes external stimuli and sends signals throughout the body. The **central nervous system (CNS)** consists of the brain and spinal cord. It is where information is processed and stored. The **peripheral nervous system (PNS)** transmits information throughout the body using electrical signals.

   **Nerve cells**, or **neurons**, communicate through electrical impulses and allow the body to process and respond to stimuli. **Neurotransmitters**, such as serotonin, dopamine, and histamines, are molecules that carry communication between nerves. Many medications act by mimicking neurotransmitters (e.g., opioids) or by altering their levels (e.g., selective serotonin reuptake inhibitors).

 **HELPFUL HINT**

Serotonin syndrome is a set of symptoms (including fever, fast heart rate, and agitation) caused by excess serotonin. It may occur with the use of any serotonergic drug but is more common when multiple serotonergic drugs are combined.

The **autonomic nervous system** controls involuntary actions that occur in the body, such as respiration, heartbeat, digestive processes, and more. The **somatic nervous system** is responsible for the body's ability to control skeletal muscles and voluntary movement as well as some involuntary reflexes.

The autonomic nervous system is further broken down into the **sympathetic nervous system** and **parasympathetic nervous system**. The sympathetic nervous system is responsible for the body's reaction to stress. It induces a "fight-or-flight" response that increases heart rate and blood pressure. In contrast, the parasympathetic nervous system is stimulated by the body's need for rest or recovery.

**Parasympathomimetic drugs** mimic acetylcholine, a neurotransmitter, and activate the parasympathetic nervous system. Nicotine is a naturally occurring parasympathetic compound.

Many common nervous system disorders are caused by chronic degeneration of nervous system tissue. Disruptions in hormone levels, electrical activity, or blood flow in the brain can also cause neurological symptoms that can signal the following conditions:

- **Mental health conditions** may be treated with medications, including anxiety, depression, bipolar disorder, schizophrenia, attention deficit hyperactivity disorder (ADHD), and post-traumatic stress disorder (PTSD).

- **Migraines** are intense headaches accompanied by nausea and light sensitivity.

- **Seizure** is caused by abnormal electrical discharges in the brain that disrupt brain function and may cause convulsions. **Epilepsy** is a condition characterized by recurrent seizures.

- **Alzheimer's disease** is characterized by the loss of memory and deteriorating cognitive function, usually later in life, due to the degeneration of neurons in the brain.

- Other degenerative nerve diseases include **multiple sclerosis (MS)**, **amyotrophic lateral sclerosis (ALS)**, and **Parkinson's disease**.

- **Stroke**, or **cardiovascular accident (CVA)**, occurs when a blood vessel in the brain ruptures or is blocked. The resulting lack of oxygen to the brain can result in significant brain damage or death.

- **Peripheral neuropathy** is impairment of the peripheral nerves. It is often caused by diabetes (diabetic neuropathy).

 **HELPFUL HINT**

Sympathomimetic drugs mimic adrenaline (epinephrine) and stimulate the autonomic nervous system. They are used for shock, allergic reactions, and cardiac arrest.

## TABLE 1.6. Antidepressants

| DRUG CLASS | COMMON DRUGS | ADVERSE REACTIONS AND INTERACTIONS |
|---|---|---|
| dopamine/norepinephrine-reuptake inhibitors | bupropion (Wellbutrin, Zyban) | |
| selective serotonin reuptake inhibitors (SSRIs) | sertraline (Zoloft), escitalopram (Lexapro), citalopram (Celexa), trazodone (Desyrel), fluoxetine (Prozac), paroxetine (Paxil) | **BBW:** increased risk of suicidal thoughts/behaviors <br> **ADR:** insomnia, headache, agitation, dizziness, drowsiness, dry mouth, nausea, vomiting <br> **Interactions:** MAOIs |
| serotonin-norepinephrine reuptake inhibitors (SNRIs) | duloxetine (Cymbalta), venlafaxine (Effexor) | |
| tricyclic antidepressants | amitriptyline (Amitid, Amitril, Elavil, Endep), nortriptyline (Pamelor) | |

**BBW:** black box warning
**ADR:** adverse drug reactions

## TABLE 1.7. Nervous System Medications

| MEDICATION | COMMON BRAND NAMES | ADVERSE REACTIONS AND INTERACTIONS |
|---|---|---|
| **ANTICONVULSANTS (*ALSO INDICATED FOR MOOD STABILIZATION): *SEIZURES, NERVE PAIN*** | | |
| gabapentin | Gralise, Neurontin | **ADR:** drowsiness, dizziness, edema, angioedema (pregabalin), suicidal thoughts, emotional changes <br> **Interactions:** alcohol, other CNS depressants |
| pregabalin | Lyrica | |
| levetiracetam | Keppra, Roweepra, Spritam | |
| lamotrigine* | Lamictal, Subvenite | **BBW:** skin rashes <br> **ADR:** dizziness, headache, nausea, visual disturbances <br> **Interactions:** other anticonvulsants, other CNS depressants, hormonal contraceptives <br> **Pregnancy:** Category D (carbamazepine) |
| carbamazepine* | Carbatrol, Epitol, Equetro, Tegretol | |
| topiramate | Topamax | **ADR:** drowsiness, dizziness, cognitive problems, tingling, anorexia <br> **Interactions:** other anticonvulsants, other CNS depressants <br> **Pregnancy:** Category D |
| valproate (divalproex)* | Depakote | **BBW:** hepatotoxicity <br> **ADR:** drowsiness, dizziness, headache, nausea and vomiting, visual disturbances <br> **Interactions:** other anticonvulsants, other CNS depressants <br> **Pregnancy:** Category D |

*continued on next page*

## TABLE 1.7. Nervous System Medications *(continued)*

| MEDICATION | COMMON BRAND NAMES | ADVERSE REACTIONS AND INTERACTIONS |
|---|---|---|
| **ANTICONVULSANTS (*ALSO INDICATED FOR MOOD STABILIZATION): *SEIZURES, NERVE PAIN*** | | |
| phenytoin | Dilantin | **ADR:** visual disturbances, slurred speech, decreased coordination, confusion<br>**Interactions:** oral contraceptives (reduces efficacy), some anticoagulants, statins<br>**Pregnancy:** Category D |
| **ATYPICAL ANTIPSYCHOTICS: *MOOD DISORDERS, SCHIZOPHRENIA*** | | |
| quetiapine fumarate | Seroquel | **BBW:** increased risk of suicidal thoughts/behaviors<br>**ADR:** drowsiness, dry mouth, dizziness, weakness, movement disorders |
| aripiprazole | Abilify | |
| risperidone | Perseris, Risperdal | |
| **TREATMENT FOR ADHD (†DRUG ALSO INDICATED FOR HYPERTENSION)** | | |
| amphetamine and dextroamphetamine | Adderall | **BBW:** potential for abuse/dependence<br>**ADR:** insomnia, headache, fast heartbeat, mood changes, decreased appetite, vomiting, dry mouth<br>**Interactions:** MAOIs |
| methylphenidate | Ritalin | |
| dexmethylphenidate | Focalin | |
| lisdexamfetamine | Vyvanse | |
| clonidine† | Catapres, Duraclon, Kapvay | **ADR:** drowsiness, headache, fatigue, dizziness, dry mouth, skin rash<br>**Interactions:** other CNS depressants |
| guanfacine† | Intuniv | |
| atomoxetine | Strattera | **BBW:** increased risk of suicidal thoughts/behaviors<br>**ADR:** headache, insomnia, dry mouth, nausea, skin rash<br>**Interactions:** MAOIs |
| **BENZODIAZEPINES: *ANXIETY, SEIZURES, MUSCLE SPASMS, INSOMNIA, ALCOHOL WITHDRAWAL*** | | |
| alprazolam | Xanax | **BBW:** risk of respiratory depression and death when used with opioids; risk of abuse/dependence<br>**ADR:** drowsiness, sedation, fatigue, memory impairment<br>**Interactions:** alcohol, other CNS depressants |
| clonazepam | Klonopin | |
| lorazepam | Ativan | |
| diazepam | Diastat, Valium, Valtoco | |
| temazepam | Restoril | |

| MEDICATION | COMMON BRAND NAMES | ADVERSE REACTIONS AND INTERACTIONS |
|---|---|---|
| **NONSTEROIDAL ANTI-INFLAMMATORY DRUGS (NSAIDS):** *PAIN, FEVER* | | |
| ibuprofen | Advil, Motrin | **BBW:** cardiovascular thrombotic events, GI bleeding<br>**ADR:** abdominal pain, diarrhea, upset stomach<br>**Pregnancy:** Category D (> 30 weeks) |
| naproxen | Aleve | |
| diclofenac | Cambia, Zipsor, Zorvolex | |
| celecoxib | Celebrex | |
| meloxicam | Mobic | |
| **OPIOIDS:** *PAIN* | | |
| acetaminophen and hydrocodone | Norco, Vicodin, Lortab | **BBW:** addiction, misuse, and abuse; respiratory depression; accidental ingestion; neonatal opioid withdrawal syndrome; risk from use with other CNS depressants<br>**ADR:** constipation, light-headedness, dizziness, nausea and vomiting<br>**Interactions:** MAOI, serotonergic drugs, alcohol, other CNS depressants<br>**Counseling:** may impair the ability to perform potentially hazardous activities |
| tramadol | Ultram | |
| oxycodone | Xtampza, OxyContin | |
| hydrocodone | Hysingla, Zohydro | |
| morphine | Arymo, Duramorph, Infumorph, Kadian, Mitigo, MS Contin | |
| **OTHER ANALGESICS:** *PAIN, FEVER* | | |
| acetaminophen | Tylenol | **BBW:** hepatotoxicity<br>**ADR:** nausea and vomiting, lightheadedness (butalbital), sedation (butalbital)<br>**Contraindications:** hepatic impairment |
| butalbital and acetaminophen | Allzital, Bupap | |
| **TREATMENT FOR PARKINSON DISEASE** | | |
| ropinirole | Requip | **ADR:** drowsiness, dizziness, hypotension, nausea, vomiting<br>**Interactions:** MAOIs (carbidopa and levodopa) |
| pramipexole | Mirapex | |
| carbidopa and levodopa | Duopa, Rytary, Sinemet | |
| **TREATMENT FOR ALZHEIMER'S DISEASE** | | |
| donepezil | Aricept | **ADR:** nausea, diarrhea, insomnia, mood changes |
| memantine | Namenda | |
| **OTHER PSYCHIATRIC DRUGS** | | |
| buspirone<br>*generalized anxiety disorder* | Buspar | **ADR:** dizziness, drowsiness<br>**Interactions:** alcohol |

*continued on next page*

## TABLE 1.7. Nervous System Medications *(continued)*

| MEDICATION | COMMON BRAND NAMES | ADVERSE REACTIONS AND INTERACTIONS |
|---|---|---|
| **OTHER PSYCHIATRIC DRUGS** | | |
| mirtazapine *mood disorders* | Remeron | **BBW**: increased risk of suicidal thoughts/behaviors<br>**ADR**: drowsiness, dry mouth, weight gain, constipation<br>**Interactions**: alcohol, other CNS depressants |
| lithium *bipolar disorder* | Lithobid | **BBW**: close monitoring required to prevent toxicity<br>**ADR**: tremor, frequent urination, thirst, nausea<br>**Interactions**: NSAIDs<br>**Pregnancy**: Category D |
| **MISCELLANEOUS** | | |
| zolpidem *sleep disorders* | Ambien | **BBW**: complex sleep behaviors<br>**ADR**: headache, drowsiness, dizziness<br>**Interactions**: other CNS depressants |
| sumatriptan *migraine or cluster headache (acute)* | Imitrex | **ADR**: tingling, dizziness<br>**Interactions**: other triptans, ergot-containing drugs<br>**Contraindications**: MAOI use |
| latanoprost *elevated intraocular pressure* | Xalatan, Xelpros | **ADR**: pain, stinging, or redness in eyes<br>**Counseling**: Wait 15 minutes after application to insert contact lenses. |
| brimonidine *rosacea, elevated intraocular pressure* | Mirvaso | **ADR** (topical): flushing, redness<br>**ADR** (ophthalmic): dry mouth; pain, stinging, or redness in eyes |

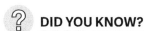 **DID YOU KNOW?**

Memory B cells are the underlying mechanisms behind vaccines, which introduce a harmless version of a pathogen into the body to activate the body's adaptive immune response.

## QUICK REVIEW QUESTIONS

13. Which of the following would be prescribed for a patient to slow the progression of Alzheimer's disease?

    A) donepezil

    B) ropinirole

    C) diazepam

    D) benazepril

14. Which drug class suffix refers to benzodiazepines?

    A) –*artan*

    B) –*pam*

    C) –*ine*

    D) –*olol*

**15.** Which auxiliary label should be affixed to a prescription bottle of buspirone?

**A)** Do not eat grapefruit or drink grapefruit juice while taking this medication.

**B)** Medication should be taken with plenty of water.

**C)** Do not take this drug if you become pregnant.

**D)** May cause drowsiness.

## The Immune System

The human **immune system** protects the body against bacteria and viruses that cause disease. The immune system includes both innate and adaptive systems. The **innate immune system** includes nonspecific defenses that work against a wide range of infectious agents. These nonspecific defenses include barriers to entry (e.g., skin), inflammation, and white blood cells (WBCs).

The **adaptive immune system** "learns" to respond only to specific invaders. The adaptive immune system relies on molecules called **antigens** that appear on the surface of pathogens to which the system has previously been exposed. **T cells** and **B cells** are activated by these antigens and destroy the invading cells. During an infection, **memory B cells** specific to an antigen are created, allowing the immune system to respond more quickly if the infection appears again.

Immune system disorders include autoimmune diseases, cancers, and infections. **Infections** can be caused by many different infectious agents, each of which are treated with a different type of medication.

### TABLE 1.8. Infectious Agents

| AGENT | DESCRIPTION | COMMON INFECTIONS | TREATMENT |
|-------|-------------|-------------------|-----------|
| **Bacteria** | single-celled prokaryotic organisms | strep throat, urinary tract infections, wound infections, many food-borne illnesses | antibiotics |
| Viruses | composed of a nucleic acid (DNA or RNA) wrapped in a protein capsid; they invade host cells and hijack cell machinery to reproduce | varicella (chicken pox), herpes zoster (shingles), herpes simplex virus, influenza, human immunodeficiency virus (HIV) | antivirals |
| Protozoa | single-celled eukaryotic organisms | giardia (an intestinal infection), trichomoniasis (a vaginal infection) | antiprotozoal drugs |
| Fungi | group of eukaryotic organisms that includes yeasts, molds, and mushrooms | athlete's foot, ringworm, oral and vaginal yeast infections | antifungals |
| Parasite | organism that lives in or on the human body and uses its resources | worms (e.g., tapeworms), flukes, lice, ticks | antiparasitic drugs |

- The immune system of individuals with an **autoimmune disease** will attack healthy tissues. Autoimmune diseases (and the tissues they attack) include:
- psoriasis (skin)

- rheumatoid arthritis (joints)
- multiple sclerosis (nerve cells)
- lupus (kidneys, lungs, and skin)
- **Allergies** are intense reactions by the immune system to harmless particles (e.g., dust, dog hair). The overreaction of the immune system can be mild (runny nose and watery eyes) or life-threatening (anaphylactic shock).
- Immune system cancers include **Hodgkin lymphoma** and **leukemia**.

 **HELPFUL HINT**

Histamines are biological molecules that mediate immune response and act as neurotransmitters. Many OTC allergy medications contain antihistamines to block histamine activity. Antihistamines can also be used as sedatives, antiemetics, and antipsychotics.

## TABLE 1.9. Antibiotics

| ANTIBIOTIC CLASS | COMMON DRUGS | ADVERSE REACTIONS AND INTERACTIONS |
|---|---|---|
| penicillins | amoxicillin (Augmentin), penicillin | |
| macrolides | azithromycin (Zithromax), clarithromycin, erythromycin | |
| tetracyclines | doxycycline, tetracycline | |
| lincosamide | clindamycin (Cleocin) | **BBW:** tendon rupture (fluroquinolones) **ADR:** diarrhea, nausea, photosensitivity (tetracyclines), tooth discoloration (tetracyclines) **Interactions:** anticoagulants, antidiabetics |
| cephalosporin | cefdinir, cephalexin (Keflex) | |
| fluoroquinolones (quinolones) | ciprofloxacin, levofloxacin (Levaquin), moxifloxacin (Avelox), ofloxacin (Floxin) | |
| sulfonamide | trimethoprim-sulfamethoxazole, co-trimoxazole (Bactrim) | |
| N/A | nitrofurantoin *urinary tract infections* | |
| aminoglycosides | gentamicin (Garamycin), tobramycin (Tobrex) | **BBW:** nephrotoxicity and neurotoxicity **ADR:** respiratory depression, lethargy, confusion, visual disturbances |
| N/A | metronidazole (Flagyl) *bacterial and protozoal infections* | **ADR:** headache, nausea, vaginitis **Contraindications:** alcohol use |

**BBW:** black box warning
**ADR:** adverse drug reactions

## TABLE 1.10. Immune Medications

| MEDICATION | COMMON BRAND NAMES | INDICATIONS | ADVERSE REACTIONS AND INTERACTIONS |
|---|---|---|---|
| **ANTIVIRALS** | | | |
| valacyclovir | Valtrex | herpes zoster | **ADR:** headache, nausea, abdominal pain |
| oseltamivir | Tamiflu | influenza | |
| acyclovir | Zovirax | herpes simplex virus, herpes zoster, varicella | |
| **CORTICOSTEROIDS** | | | |
| fluticasone | Flonase (nasal), Flovent (oral inhalant) | asthma, COPD (oral inhalation) allergies (nasal) dermatitis (topical) inflammation, autoimmune conditions (oral tablet) | **ADR** (nasal/oral inhalation): headache, nasal/throat irritation, nose bleed, cough, worsening of infections<br>**ADR** (oral tablet): fluid retention, hyper/hypoglycemia, hypertension, changes in behavior/mood, weight gain, worsening of infections<br>**Interactions** (oral tablet): antidiabetics, anticoagulants, oral contraceptives, NSAIDs |
| prednisone | Sterapred (oral tablet) | | |
| triamcinolone | Nasacort (nasal) | | |
| prednisolone | Millipred (oral tablet), Orapred ODT (oral tablet) | | |
| beclomethasone | QVAR RediHaler (oral inhalant), QNASL (nasal) | | |
| hydrocortisone | Cortaid (topical) | | |
| methylprednisolone | Medrol (oral tablet) | | |
| budesonide | Rhinocort (nasal), Entocort (oral tablet) | | |
| mometasone | Asmanex (oral inhalant) | | |
| **HISTAMINE H1 ANTAGONISTS** | | | |
| loratadine | Alavert, Claritin | allergies | **ADR:** drowsiness, nasal/throat irritation, dry mouth, muscle pain<br>**Interactions:** other CNS depressants |
| cetirizine | Zyrtec | | |
| levocetirizine | Xyzal Allergy | | |
| promethazine | Phenergan, Promethegan | allergies, nausea/vomiting, motion sickness | |
| hydroxyzine | Vistaril | anxiety, allergies, nausea/vomiting | |
| meclizine | Dramamine | motion sickness | |

*continued on next page*

## TABLE 1.10. Immune Medications (*continued*)

| MEDICATION | COMMON BRAND NAMES | INDICATIONS | ADVERSE REACTIONS AND INTERACTIONS |
|---|---|---|---|
| **IMMUNOSUPPRESSANTS** | | | |
| methotrexate | Otrexup, Rasuvo, Trexall, Xatmep | cancer, arthritis, psoriasis | **BBW:** fetal toxicity, severe or fatal adverse reactions<br>**ADR:** nausea, fatigue, stomach upset, increased risk of infection<br>**Pregnancy:** Category X |
| adalimumab | Humira | Crohn's disease, rheumatoid arthritis, psoriasis, ulcerative colitis | **BBW:** risk of serious infection<br>**ADR:** infection, headache, rash |
| **MISCELLANEOUS** | | | |
| hydroxychloroquine | Plaquenil | lupus, malaria, rheumatoid arthritis | **ADR:** blurred vision, blistering or peeling of skin, dizziness, nausea, vomiting<br>**Interactions:** digoxin, insulin, antidiabetic drugs, antiepileptics |
| fluconazole | Diflucan | fungal infections | **ADR:** headache, nausea, abdominal pain<br>**Interactions:** antidiabetics, anticoagulants, benzodiazepines |
| **BBW:** black box warning<br>**ADR:** adverse drug reactions | | | |

## QUICK REVIEW QUESTIONS

**16.** Patients who have previously had an allergic reaction to azithromycin should have a note in their profile about an allergy to which class of antibiotics?

**A)** macrolides

**B)** tetracyclines

**C)** quinolones

**D)** penicillins

**17.** Which of the following medications is an immunosuppressant?

**A)** valacyclovir

**B)** methotrexate

**C)** cefdinir

**D)** carbamazepine

## The Musculoskeletal System

The skeletal system is made up of over 200 different **bones**, which are stiff connective tissues in the human body. The bones have many functions, including:

- protecting internal organs
- synthesizing blood cells
- storing necessary minerals
- providing the muscular system with leverage to create movement

The point at which a bone is attached to another bone is called a **joint**. Various connective tissues join the parts of the skeleton together to other systems, including ligaments, tendons, and cartilage.

The primary function of the **muscular system** is movement: muscles contract and relax, resulting in motion. The muscular system consists of three types of muscle: cardiac, visceral, and skeletal.

- **Cardiac muscle** is only found in the heart. It contracts involuntarily, creating the heartbeat and pumping blood.
- **Visceral**, or **smooth**, **muscle** tissue is found in many of the body's essential organs, including the stomach and intestines. It contracts involuntarily to move nutrients, blood, and other substances throughout the body.
- **Skeletal muscle** is responsible for voluntary movement and, as the name suggests, is linked to the skeletal system.

Most musculoskeletal system disorders are caused by the degeneration of tissue or damage to muscles or bones from trauma.

- **Arthritis** is inflammation in joints.
- **Gout** is inflammation and pain in joints caused by a buildup of uric acid.
- **Osteoporosis** is poor bone mineral density due to the loss or lack of production of calcium content in bone cells, which makes bones more likely to fracture.
- **Osteomyelitis** is an infection in the bone.
- **Muscular dystrophy (MD)** is a genetically inherited condition that results in progressive muscle wasting, which limits movement and can cause respiratory and cardiovascular difficulties.
- Muscle **cramps** are involuntary muscle contractions (or **spasms**) that cause intense pain.

CONTINUE

## TABLE 1.11. Musculoskeletal Medications

| MEDICATION | COMMON BRAND NAMES | ADVERSE REACTIONS AND INTERACTIONS |
|---|---|---|
| **MUSCLE RELAXANTS AND ANTISPASMODICS:** *MUSCLE SPASM* | | |
| cyclobenzaprine | Flexeril | **BBW:** abrupt discontinuation (baclofen)<br>**ADR:** drowsiness, dizziness, dry mouth, nausea and vomiting<br>**Interactions:** alcohol, other CNS depressants, MAOIs, serotonergic drugs<br>**Contraindications:** use of MAOIs (cyclobenzaprine), use of ciprofloxacin or fluvoxamine (tizanidine) |
| tizanidine | Zanaflex | |
| baclofen | Gablofen, Lioresal, Ozobax | |
| methocarbamol | Robaxin | |
| **MISCELLANEOUS** | | |
| alendronate<br>*osteoporosis* | Binosto, Fosamax | **ADR:** headache, upset stomach, musculoskeletal pain<br>**Interactions:** calcium supplements, antacids, NSAIDs<br>**Counseling:** Take with water 30 minutes before first food of the day. |

**BBW:** black box warning
**ADR:** adverse drug reactions

## QUICK REVIEW QUESTIONS

**18.** A patient presents a new prescription for cyclobenzaprine. The pharmacy technician should alert the pharmacist to a potential interaction if the patient is currently prescribed which of the following medications?

**A)** Nexium

**B)** Januvia

**C)** Zoloft

**D)** Ortho Tri-Cyclen

**19.** Which auxiliary label should be affixed to a prescription bottle of alendronate?

**A)** Do not take antacids within one hour of this medication.

**B)** Do not eat grapefruit or drink grapefruit juice while taking this medication.

**C)** Do not take this drug if you become pregnant.

**D)** Do not drink alcoholic beverages while taking this medication.

## The Digestive System

The **digestive system** is responsible for the breakdown and absorption of food necessary to power the body. The digestive system starts at the **mouth**. Chewed and lubricated food travels from the mouth through the **esophagus**, which leads to the **stomach**. In the stomach, food is mixed with powerful acidic liquid for further digestion. The resulting **chyme** travels to the **small intestine**, where nutrients are absorbed.

The small intestine then transports food to the **large intestine**, which absorbs water and produces feces. At the end of the large intestine are the **rectum** and **anus**, which are responsible for the storage and removal of feces.

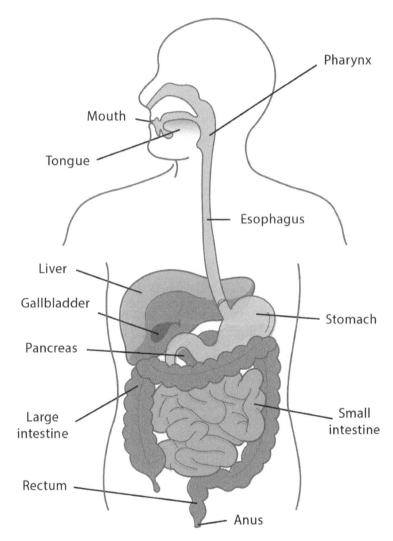

*Figure 1.7. The Digestive System*

The digestive system also includes accessory organs that aid in digestion:

- **salivary glands**: produce saliva, which begins the process of breaking down starches and fats

- **liver**: produces bile, which helps break down fat in the small intestine (The liver also plays an important role in the metabolism of many proteins and carbohydrates.)
- **gallbladder**: stores bile
- **pancreas**: produces pancreatic juice, which neutralizes the acidity of chyme and digestive enzymes

    Common gastrointestinal disorders include infections, autoimmune disorders, and liver disease.

- **Heartburn** occurs when stomach acid moves into the esophagus.
- **Food poisoning** occurs when an acute infection (bacterial or viral) affects the lining of the digestive system and the resulting immune response triggers the body to void the contents of the digestive system.
- **Irritable bowel syndrome (IBS)** refers to recurrent abdominal pain, bloating, diarrhea, or constipation.
- **Crohn's disease** is an inflammatory bowel disorder that occurs when the immune system attacks the digestive system.
- **Cirrhosis** is a chronic disease in which the liver has permanent scarring and loses cells, impairing normal functioning. The most common cause of cirrhosis is alcohol abuse.

    Many of the drugs used for the digestive system are available OTC and may alleviate digestive symptoms developed from heartburn, diet, gas, nausea, and food poisoning.

- **Antacids** are used primarily for heartburn but also as a calcium supplement. Some common brands of antacids are Tums and Rolaids.
- **Antidiarrheal drugs** help reduce or stop diarrhea. A common OTC antidiarrheal drug is loperamide (Imodium A-D).
- **Laxatives** treat constipation. OTC laxatives include bisacodyl (Dulcolax), polyethylene glycol (MiraLAX), and sennoside (Milk of Magnesia, Ex-Lax).
- **Stool softeners**, like docusate sodium (Colace), soften the stool and do not cause as much urgency and cramping as laxatives do.
- **Fiber supplements**, such as methylcellulose (Metamucil), help to keep the body regular and prevent constipation.

## TABLE 1.12. Digestive Medications

| MEDICATION | COMMON BRAND NAMES | ADVERSE REACTIONS AND INTERACTIONS |
|---|---|---|
| **ANTIEMETICS: *NAUSEA AND VOMITING*** | | |
| ondansetron | Zofran | **ADR:** headache, constipation, and diarrhea<br>**Interactions:** serotonergic drugs |

| MEDICATION | COMMON BRAND NAMES | ADVERSE REACTIONS AND INTERACTIONS |
|---|---|---|
| prochlorperazine | Compro | **ADR:** drowsiness, dizziness, blurred vision, hypotension<br>**Interactions:** other CNS depressants |
| doxylamine and pyridoxine | Diclegis | **ADR:** drowsiness<br>**Interactions:** other CNS depressants |
| **HISTAMINE H2 ANTAGONIST: *HEARTBURN, GERD*** | | |
| ranitidine | Zantac | **ADR:** headache, constipation, diarrhea, nausea, vomiting<br>**Interactions:** warfarin |
| famotidine | Pepcid | |
| **PROTON PUMP INHIBITORS: *HEARTBURN, GERD*** | | |
| omeprazole | Prilosec | **ADR:** headache, abdominal pain, nausea, diarrhea, vomiting<br>**Interactions:** digoxin, clopidogrel, benzodiazepines, warfarin |
| pantoprazole | Protonix | |
| esomeprazole | Nexium | |
| lansoprazole | Prevacid | |
| **SUPPLEMENTS** | | |
| potassium | | **ADR:** nausea, vomiting, flatulence, abdominal pain/discomfort, and diarrhea<br>**Interactions:** potassium-sparing diuretics |
| ergocalciferol (vitamin D) | Deltalin, Drisdol, Ergocal | none |
| ferrous sulfate (iron) | | **BBW:** accidental overdose in children<br>**ADR:** darkened stool, abdominal pain, heartburn, constipation, nausea, vomiting |
| folic acid | FA-8 | none |
| cyanocobalamin (vitamin B-12) | | **ADR:** headache, infection, weakness |
| **MISCELLANEOUS** | | |
| dicyclomine<br>*irritable bowel syndrome* | Bentyl | **ADR:** dry mouth, nausea, vomiting, constipation, dizziness, blurred vision<br>**Interactions:** other anticholinergics<br>**Counseling:** may impair the ability to perform potentially hazardous activities |
| phentermine<br>*obesity* | Adipex-P, Lomaira | **ADR:** restlessness, dizziness, dry mouth<br>**Interactions:** alcohol, MAOI, insulin<br>**Pregnancy:** Category X<br>**Counseling:** may impair the ability to perform potentially hazardous activities |

**BBW:** black box warning
**ADR:** adverse drug reactions

## QUICK REVIEW QUESTIONS

**20.** Antiemetics are taken to prevent

**A)** vomiting.

**B)** diarrhea.

**C)** constipation.

**D)** gas.

**21.** Which of the following medications is a proton pump inhibitor?

**A)** misoprostol

**B)** famotidine

**C)** sucralfate

**D)** pantoprazole

## The Endocrine System

The endocrine system is made up of **glands** that regulate numerous processes throughout the body by secreting chemical messengers called **hormones**. Hormones regulate a wide variety of bodily processes, including metabolism, growth and development, sexual reproduction, the sleep-wake cycle, and hunger. Important endocrine organs and their functions are below.

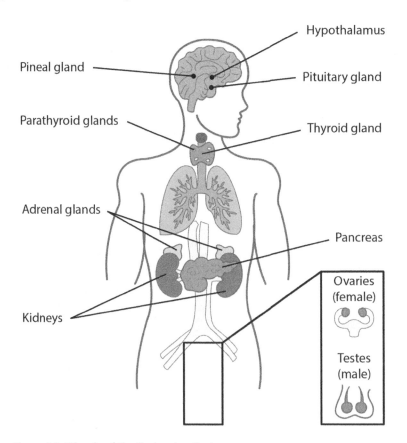

*Figure 1.8. Glands of the Endocrine System*

- The **pancreas** produces insulin and glucagon, which regulate blood sugar levels.

- The **thyroid gland** controls metabolism.
- The **pituitary gland** controls growth and basic functions, such as temperature and blood pressure.
- The **adrenal glands** produce adrenaline (epinephrine).
- The **parathyroid gland** controls calcium and phosphate levels in the blood.
- The **ovaries** (female) and **testes** (male) produce hormones related to sexual functioning.

Disruptions in hormone production can affect multiple systems throughout the body.

- **Diabetes mellitus** is a metabolic disorder that affects the body's ability to produce and use **insulin,** a hormone that regulates the cellular uptake of glucose (sugar). Diabetes mellitus is classified as type 1 or type 2.
- **Hypothyroidism** occurs when insufficient thyroxine is produced and can result in fatigue, weight gain, and cold intolerance.
- **Hyperthyroidism** occurs when too much thyroxine is produced and can cause anxiety, mood swings, weight loss, and palpitations. Grave's disease is a specific cause of hyperthyroidism common in women over 40.
- **Adrenal insufficiency** (Addison's disease) is the chronic underproduction of steroids.
- **Cushing syndrome** is caused by exposure to high cortisol levels over an extended period of time due to overproduction of cortisol from the adrenal glands.
- **Hypercalcemia** is a treatable condition in which the parathyroid glands become overactive, causing the blood to have a high calcium level.

 **HELPFUL HINT**

One of the most prescribed medications in the US is levothyroxine (Synthroid), a manufactured form of the hormone thyroxine. It is prescribed for patients with underactive thyroids.

## TABLE 1.13. Endocrine Medications

| MEDICATION | COMMON BRAND NAMES | ADVERSE REACTIONS AND INTERACTIONS |
| --- | --- | --- |
| **ANTIDIABETICS: *DIABETES*** | | |
| metformin | Fortamet, Glucophage | |
| glipizide | Glucotrol | |
| glimepiride | Amaryl | |
| sitagliptin | Januvia | **ADR:** hypoglycemia, diarrhea, nausea, headache |
| pioglitazone | Actos | **Interactions:** alcohol, miconazole (glimepiride) |
| liraglutide | Saxenda, Victoza | **Counseling:** Take with food (metformin); Take 30 minutes before food (glipizide). |
| glyburide | Glynase | |
| canagliflozin | Invokana | |
| linagliptin | Tradjenta | |
| sitagliptin and metformin | Janumet | |

*continued on next page*

## TABLE 1.13. Endocrine Medications (continued)

| MEDICATION | COMMON BRAND NAMES | ADVERSE REACTIONS AND INTERACTIONS |
|---|---|---|
| **INSULINS: DIABETES** | | |
| insulin glargine | Lantus | **ADR:** hypoglycemia, injection site reactions<br>**Interactions:** other insulin products |
| insulin aspart | Fiasp, Novolog | |
| insulin human (insulin regular) | Humulin, Novolin | |
| insulin detemir | Levemir | |
| insulin lispro | ADMELOG, Humalog | |
| **MISCELLANEOUS** | | |
| Levothyroxine (synthetic thyroxine)<br>*hypothyroidism* | Levoxyl, Synthroid, Tirosint, Unithroid | **BBW:** weight reduction<br>**ADR:** dysrhythmias, trouble breathing, headache, nervousness, irritability, weight loss<br>**Interactions:** iron supplement, calcium supplement, antacids<br>**Counseling:** Take with water 30 minutes before eating. |
| propylthiouracil<br>*hyperthyroidism* | | **BBW:** hepatotoxicity<br>**ADR:** upset stomach, nausea, vomiting, headache, drowsiness, hair loss<br>**Interactions:** anticoagulants, beta blockers<br>**Pregnancy:** Category D |
| **BBW:** black box warning<br>**ADR:** adverse drug reactions | | |

## QUICK REVIEW QUESTIONS

**22.** Which of the following is a common adverse reaction to levothyroxine?

    **A)** drowsiness

    **B)** constipation

    **C)** weight loss

    **D)** dry mouth

**23.** Which of the following is NOT a type of manufactured insulin?

    **A)** lispro

    **B)** detemir

    **C)** glargine

    **D)** dulaglutide

# The Urinary System

The **urinary system** excretes water and waste from the body and is crucial for maintaining the balance of water and salt in the blood (also called electrolyte balance). The main organs of the urinary system are the **kidneys**, which perform several important functions:

- filter waste from the blood

- maintain the electrolyte balance in the blood

- regulate blood volume, pressure, and pH

**Nephrons** in the kidneys filter the blood and excrete the waste products as **urine**. Urine then passes through the ureters into the urinary bladder and exits through the **urethra**.

Common urinary system conditions that may require medication include infections, incontinence, and fluid/electrolyte imbalances.

- **Urinary incontinence**—loss of bladder control—is a common problem, especially in women over 40, and can range from slight to severe incontinence.

- **Renal calculi** (kidney stones) are hardened mineral deposits that form in the kidneys and cause pain and urinary symptoms.

- **Urinary tract infections (UTIs)** can occur in the lower urinary tract (bladder and urethra) or in the upper urinary tract (kidneys and ureters).

- **Renal failure** is the loss of kidney function that leads to buildup of waste in the bloodstream. It can be acute or chronic.

 **HELPFUL HINT**

Diuretics alter the function of nephrons, causing the kidneys to absorb and excrete more water. They are used to treat edema (swelling due to fluid buildup) caused by heart, lung, or kidney disease.

## TABLE 1.14. Urinary Medications

| MEDICATION | COMMON BRAND NAMES | ADVERSE REACTIONS AND INTERACTIONS |
|---|---|---|
| **DIURETICS: *HYPERTENSION, EDEMA*** | | |
| hydrochlorothiazide | Microzide | |
| furosemide | Lasix | |
| spironolactone | Aldactone, CaroSpir | **BBW:** fluid/electrolyte loss (furosemide), pregnancy (lisinopril) |
| chlorthalidone | | **ADR:** hypotension, weakness, dizziness, blurred vision |
| hydrochlorothiazide and triamterene | Dyazide, Maxzide | **Interactions:** alcohol, other antihypertensive drugs, NSAIDs |
| hydrochlorothiazide and lisinopril | Zestoretic | |

*continued on next page*

| TABLE 1.14. Urinary Medications *(continued)* | | |
|---|---|---|
| **MEDICATION** | **COMMON BRAND NAMES** | **ADVERSE REACTIONS AND INTERACTIONS** |
| **TREATMENT OF OVERACTIVE BLADDER** | | |
| oxybutynin | Ditropan XL, Gelnique, Oxytrol | **ADR:** constipation, dry mouth, dizziness, drowsiness **Interactions:** anticholinergic drugs |
| trospium | Trosec | |
| mirabegron | Myrbetriq | **ADR:** hypertension, nose and throat irritation, dry mouth, headache **Interactions:** digoxin |
| **MISCELLANEOUS** | | |
| allopurinol *gout* | Lopurin, Zyloprim, Aloprim | **ADR:** rash, nausea, vomiting, drowsiness **Interactions:** anticoagulants **Counseling:** may impair the ability to perform potentially hazardous activities |
| **BBW:** black box warning **ADR:** adverse drug reactions | | |

## QUICK REVIEW QUESTIONS

**24.** Which of the following medications may be prescribed to treat edema caused by liver failure?

**A)** spironolactone

**B)** benazepril

**C)** oxybutynin

**D)** pravastatin

**25.** Which auxiliary label should be affixed to a prescription bottle of oxybutynin?

**A)** Chew tablets before swallowing.

**B)** May cause drowsiness/dizziness.

**C)** Medication should be taken with plenty of water.

**D)** Do not take this drug if you become pregnant.

## The Reproductive System

The **male reproductive system** produces **sperm**, or male gametes, and passes them to the female reproductive system. Sperm are produced in the **testes** (also called testicles), which are housed in a sac-like external structure called the **scrotum**. During sexual stimulation, sperm mixes with fluids from the **seminal** vesicles, **prostate**, and **Cowper's gland**. The mix of fluids and sperm, called **semen**, travels through the urethra and exits the body through the **penis**, which becomes rigid during sexual arousal.

The main hormone associated with the male reproductive system is **testosterone**, which is released mainly by the testes. Testosterone is responsible for the development of the male reproductive system and male secondary sexual characteristics, including muscle development and facial hair growth.

The **female reproductive system** produces **eggs**, or female gametes, and gestates the **fetus** during pregnancy. Eggs are produced in the **ovaries** and travel through the **fallopian tubes** to the **uterus**, which is a muscular organ that houses the fetus during pregnancy. The uterine cavity is lined with a layer of blood-rich tissue called the **endometrium**. If no pregnancy occurs, the endometrium is shed monthly during **menstruation**.

**Fertilization** occurs when the egg absorbs the sperm. After fertilization now the new **zygote** implants itself in the endometrium, where it will grow and develop over thirty-eight weeks (roughly nine months). During gestation, nutrients and waste pass between the fetus and mother via the **umbilical cord**, which is attached to the **placenta**. During labor, uterine contractions push the baby through the **cervix** and out of the **vagina**.

The female reproductive cycle is controlled by several different hormones, including **estrogen** and **progesterone**.

Patients may require prescription medications to manage infections, cancers, and dysfunction of the reproductive systems.

- **Sexually transmitted infections (STIs)** occur in both males and females. Common STIs include chlamydia, gonorrhea, genital herpes, human papillomavirus (HPV), and syphilis.
- **Endometriosis** is a painful disorder in which the tissue that lines the uterus grows outside the uterus.
- **Menopause** is the natural decline in the reproduction of hormones in women, typically when they reach their forties or fifties.
- **Benign prostatic hypertrophy** (BPH) is an age-associated condition in which the prostate gland enlarges, causing urinary difficulty.
- **Erectile dysfunction** (ED) is when a man cannot achieve or keep an erection strong enough for sexual intercourse.
- **Prostate cancer** afflicts the male prostate.
- **Breast cancer**, although most common in women, can afflict men as well.

 **DID YOU KNOW?**

Most oral contraceptive pills prevent pregnancy by stopping ovulation (the release of eggs from the ovaries).

 **HELPFUL HINT**

**Alpha2-adrenergic** agonists (suffix *–ine*) act on the central nervous system and are used to treat a wide range of conditions, including BPH, hypertension, muscle spasms, and alcohol/ opioid withdrawal.

→
CONTINUE

## TABLE 1.15. Reproductive Medications

| MEDICATION | COMMON BRAND NAMES | ADVERSE REACTIONS AND INTERACTIONS |
|---|---|---|
| **CONTRACEPTIVES** | | |
| ethinyl estradiol and norethin-drone | Cyclafem 7/7/7, Femhrt, Loestrin, Ortho-Novum | **BBW:** increased risk of cardiovascular disease with smoking, increased risk of endometrial and breast cancer<br>**ADR:** nausea, vomiting, headache, menstrual irregularities, weight change, breast tenderness<br>**Interactions:** some anticonvulsants (e.g., topiramate), St. John's wort<br>**Pregnancy:** Category X |
| ethinyl estradiol and norgestimate | Ortho Tri-Cyclen, Sprintec, TriNessa | |
| ethinyl estradiol and drospirenone | Ocella, Yasmin, Zarah | |
| ethinyl estradiol and levonorgestrel | Plan B One-Step, Jolessa, Seasonique, Mirena | |
| ethinyl estradiol and desogestrel | Apri, Kariva | |
| ethinyl estradiol and etonogestrel | NuvaRing | |
| norethindrone | Camilla, Errin | |
| **HORMONES** | | |
| Estradiol (estrogen)<br>*low estrogen, osteoporosis prophylaxis, symptoms of menopause* | | **BBW:** increased risk of endometrial cancer, breast cancer, and cardiovascular disease<br>**ADR:** edema, headache, mood changes, rash, breast tenderness, nasal or throat irritation |
| Testosterone<br>*breast cancer, delayed puberty, hypogonadism* | | **BBW:** blood pressure increases, secondary exposure<br>**ADR:** hypertension, blister or irritation at application site<br>**Interactions:** anticoagulants |
| Progesterone<br>*assisted reproductive technology, amenorrhea* | Crinone, Endometrin, Prometrium | **BBW:** increased risk of breast cancer and cardiovascular disorders<br>**ADR:** edema, mood changes, nausea, breast tenderness<br>**Interactions:** anticoagulants |
| **TREATMENT OF BPH (*ALSO INDICATED FOR HYPERTENSION)** | | |
| tamsulosin | Flomax | **ADR:** orthostatic hypotension, sexual disorder, dizziness, headache |
| doxazosin* | Cardura | |
| terazosin* | | |
| finasteride | Propecia, Proscar | |

| MEDICATION | COMMON BRAND NAMES | ADVERSE REACTIONS AND INTERACTIONS |
|---|---|---|
| **TREATMENT OF ERECTILE DYSFUNCTION** | | |
| sildenafil | Revatio, Viagra | **ADR:** headache, flushing, upset stomach, abnormal vision, congestion, nausea |
| tadalafil | Cialis | **Interactions:** anti-hypertensives |
| vardenafil | Levitra | **Contraindications:** nitrate use |
| **BBW:** black box warning **ADR:** adverse drug reactions | | |

## QUICK REVIEW QUESTIONS

**26.** Which of the following is a BPH medication?

**A)** buserelin

**B)** terazosin

**C)** progesterone

**D)** clomiphene

**27.** Which OTC product may reduce the effectiveness of hormonal contraceptives?

**A)** phenylephrine

**B)** NSAIDs

**C)** iron supplements

**D)** St. John's wort

## The Integumentary System

The **integumentary system** refers to the skin (the largest organ in the body) and related structures, including the hair and nails. The **skin** is composed of three layers: the epidermis (outer layer), dermis, and hypodermis (inner layer).

The skin has several important roles. It houses nerves, and it acts as a barrier to protect the body from injury, the intrusion of foreign particles, and the loss of water and nutrients. It also produces vitamin D and helps thermoregulation.

Most integumentary disorders that require prescribed medications are bacterial, fungal, or parasitic infections. The skin can also be damaged by trauma, which may require antibiotics or analgesics.

- **Acne** is the most common skin infection. Although it is most prevalent in adolescents, acne can happen at any age.

- **Staphylococcus** (staph) **infection** is caused by an accumulation of the bacteria staphylococcus, normally found on the skin or nose. It is very contagious. **Methicillin-resilient staphylococcus aureus** (MRSA) can only be treated with certain kinds of antibiotics.

- **Fungal infections** are caused by an overgrowth of fungus. **Candida** is the most common. Symptoms include a skin rash and itching.
- **Rashes** are itchy, inflamed skin usually caused by allergic reactions.
- **Scabies** is caused by a tiny mite that burrows into the skin.
- **Rosacea** is a chronic condition that causes redness and small, pus-filled bumps on the face. It tends to affect fair-skinned women.
- **Impetigo** is a highly contagious skin infection that causes sores and is mainly seen in children.
- **Skin cancer** is caused by an abnormal growth of cells on the skin and presents in many forms.
- **Sunburns** can be very painful, cause chills or fevers, and lead to sun poisoning.

### TABLE 1.16. Integumentary Medications

| MEDICATION | COMMON BRAND NAMES | ADVERSE REACTIONS AND INTERACTIONS |
|---|---|---|
| **TOPICAL ANTIBIOTICS** | | |
| bacitracin, neomycin, and polymyxin B | Neosporin | **ADR:** burning, stinging, rash |
| mupirocin | Centany | |
| **TOPICAL ANTIFUNGALS** | | |
| miconazole | Lotrimin | **ADR:** itching, rash |
| nystatin | Nyamyc, Nystop | |
| tolnaftate | Tinactin | |
| **ADR:** adverse drug reactions | | |

## QUICK REVIEW QUESTION

**28.** Which of the following would be prescribed to treat a skin infection caused by Candida albicans?

**A)** benzocaine

**B)** anthralin

**C)** imiquimod

**D)** nystatin

## Radiopharmaceuticals

**Radiopharmaceutical drugs** have a radioactive compound and are used for diagnostic and therapeutic purposes. As with all pharmaceuticals, a standard is required for implementing and developing these drugs.

Most radiopharmaceuticals are used for diagnostic imaging, but they can also be used for chemotherapy and radiation in cancer patients. Chemotherapy radiopharmaceuticals include strontium 89 (Metastron), samarium 153 (Quadramet), and radium-223 (Xofigo) for bone cancers; radioactive iodine for thyroid cancer; and phosphorus 32 for brain tumors.

**Monoclonal antibodies**, or **radio-labeled antibodies**, are manufactured versions of immune system proteins with radioactive atoms that only attach to their target. This treatment is used for non-Hodgkin lymphoma.

## QUICK REVIEW QUESTION

29. Which of these is NOT a radiopharmaceutical?

    A) monoclonal antibodies

    B) radium 450

    C) phosphorus 32

    D) radium 223

## Drug Stability Storage

Drugs degrade over time, so manufacturers put **expiration dates** on every product to ensure that medications will work properly when taken. The expiration date is usually a month and year, and the medication is considered usable through the end of the given month. For example, if the expiration date on a drug is 7/22, the last day it should be taken is 7/31/2022.

Once a drug has been removed from its packaging for compounding or repackaging, the expiration date on the original package is no longer valid. Instead, the pharmacy calculates a **beyond-use date (BUD)** that is included on the new drug label. For repackaged non-sterile solids or liquids, the BUD is one year after the repackaging date or the original expiration date, whichever comes first.

When a medication is compounded, due to degradation it is only good for a limited amount of time. These medications will have a BUD that is specific to the product. For example, reconstituted Vancomycin must be used within 7 days. So the BUD for this compound made on 7/10/2021 would be 7/17/2021. The BUD must be included on the label for compounded medications. It is usually written as "Discard After" or "Do Not Use After."

## QUICK REVIEW QUESTION

30. On 11/3/2021, a pharmacy technician uses a bottle of amoxicillin with an expiration date of 3/31/2022 to make an oral suspension. If the oral suspension must be used within 10 days, what beyond-use date should the technician put on the label?

    A) 11/3/2021

    B) 11/13/2021

    C) 3/31/2022

    D) 4/10/2022

## Drug Storage

Drugs must be stored properly to ensure drug integrity. Factors that may influence the rate at which drugs degrade include temperature, light, air, and moisture.

Drugs should be stored at the temperature recommended by the manufacturer. The packaging will state whether a drug should be kept at **room temperature** (59°F – 86°F [15°C – 30°C]), **refrigerated** (36°F – 46°F [2°C – 8°C]), or **frozen** (–13°F – 14°F [–25° – –10°C]).

Some drugs will degrade faster when exposed to light. Light-sensitive solids are usually coated to protect them from light or are stored in opaque packaging. Light-sensitive liquids, including reconstituted drugs, should be stored in amber or opaque vials. Examples of drugs that should be protected from light include insulin, furosemide, and sumatriptan.

**HELPFUL HINT**

Common refrigerated drugs include regular insulin, reconstituted antibiotics, and some vaccines (e.g., influenza, Tdap, rotavirus).

### QUICK REVIEW QUESTION

31. A patient is picking up a prescription for amoxicillin, which the pharmacy technician has reconstituted. Where should the patient store this medication?

    A) a dry area at room temperature

    B) away from light sources

    C) a refrigerator

    D) a freezer

1.  **C)** Naloxone is an opioid antagonist. It binds to opioid receptors and prevents opioid agonists (such as morphine and oxycodone) from binding to those sites.

2.  **B)** The color of a drug does not affect its ability to treat its targeted disease or condition.

3.  **C)** Drugs do not have to have the same active ingredient to be in the same drug class since each drug is chemically different.

4.  **D)** Contraceptive failure caused by interaction between medications is an example of an adverse drug reaction of type F (failure of therapy).

5.  **A)** Omeprazole (Prilosec) can decrease the effectiveness of clopidogrel (Plavix), which is a drug-drug interaction.

6.  **C)** Metformin is an antidiabetic that should be taken with food.

7.  **A)** SL is the abbreviation for sublingual, meaning "under the tongue."

8.  **D)** ACE inhibitors, such as benazepril, fosinopril, and quinapril, have the *-pril* suffix.

9.  **C)** Vasodilators relax blood vessels, reducing the force of the heart and the pressure of the blood against the vessel walls.

10. **B)** Nitroglycerin should not be taken with erectile dysfunction medications such as tadalafil (Cialis).

11. **A)** Montelukast (Singulair) is an inhaled bronchodilator prescribed for the treatment of asthma.

12. **D)** Benzonatate should be swallowed whole to prevent numbing of the mouth and throat.

13. **A)** Donepezil is a cognition-enhancing medication used to slow the progression of Alzheimer's disease.

14. **B)** The suffix *-pam* refers to benzodiazepines.

15. **D)** Buspirone is an anti-anxiety medication that may cause drowsiness.

16. **A)** Azithromycin is a macrolide antibiotic.

17. **B)** Methotrexate is an immunosuppressant prescribed to treat cancer and some autoimmune conditions.

18. **C)** Sertraline (Zoloft) is an SSRI. Combining cyclobenzaprine and a serotonergic drug may lead to serotonin syndrome.

19. **A)** Antacids decrease the absorption of alendronate (Fosamax), so the drugs should not be taken together.

20. **A)** Antiemetics prevent nausea and vomiting.

21. **D)** Pantoprazole is a proton pump inhibitor.

22. **C)** Levothyroxine is a synthetic thyroid hormone that increases metabolism, which may result in weight loss.

23. **D)** Dulaglutide (Trulicity) is an antidiabetic, not an insulin.

24. **A)** Spironolactone is a diuretic used to treat edema caused by liver failure.

25. **B)** Oxybutynin is an anticholinergic drug that may cause drowsiness or dizziness.

26. **B)** Terazosin is an alpha-adrenergic blocker prescribed to treat benign prostatic hypertrophy or hypertension.

27. **D)** Taking St. John's wort can reduce the effectiveness of hormonal contraceptive pills.

28. **D)** Nystatin is an antifungal used to treat Candida infections.

29. **B)** Radium 450 is not a radiopharmaceutical.

30. **B)** The beyond-use date should be ten days after the solution is reconstituted, which would be 11/13/2021.

31. **C)** Reconstituted amoxicillin should be refrigerated.

# 2 | Federal Requirements

## Regulatory Agencies and Organizations

The **US Food and Drug Administration (FDA)** is part of the US Department of Health and Human Services. It approves applications for new drugs and medical devices and investigates the improper use and misbranding of agricultural goods and services used for food and drugs.

The **Drug Enforcement Agency (DEA)** is part of the US Department of Justice. The DEA enforces the Controlled Substances Act to prevent the diversion and abuse of both controlled substances and chemicals regulated by the FDA. The DEA is involved in every aspect of the handling and distribution of controlled substances and regulated chemicals.

The **Bureau of Alcohol, Tobacco, Firearms and Explosives (ATF)** is a federal organization within the US Department of Justice. The ATF combats terrorism, arson, and violent crime; it regulates alcohol, tobacco, firearms, and explosives.

The **state boards of pharmacy (BOP)** regulate, by state, the practice of pharmacy. State BOPs mainly focus on the public's health and the implementation and enforcement of state pharmacy law.

The **Centers for Medicare & Medicaid Services (CMS)** manages Medicare, Medicaid, the Children's Health Insurance Program (CHIP), and the health insurance exchanges.

The **US Pharmacopeial Convention (USP)** is a nonprofit organization that sets standards for the strength, purity, quality, and identity of medicines, dietary supplements, and food. The USP sets standards for preparing compounds.

**The Joint Commission** is a nonprofit organization whose main function is to enhance patient safety and quality of care in institutional environments. The Joint Commission accredits hospitals through yearly inspections for compliance and national patient safety goals.

The **Institute for Safe Medication Practices (ISMP)** is a nonprofit that operates a medication error reporting system and issues regular alerts for recurring medication errors.

 **HELPFUL HINT**

MedWatch is the FDA's safety and adverse event reporting program.

1. Which of the following agencies is responsible for monitoring the handling and distribution of controlled substances?

   A) Centers for Medicare & Medicaid Services

   B) Drug Enforcement Agency

   C) Food and Drug Administration

   D) state boards of pharmacy

## Controlled Substances

**Controlled substances** are drugs that are strictly regulated by the government; prescribers must follow specific rules when prescribing them that differ from non-controlled drugs. The **Controlled Substances Act (CSA)**, a federal drug policy that was passed in 1970, strictly controls the manufacture, importation, possession, use, and distribution of certain controlled substances. The substances it covers are narcotics, stimulants, depressants, hallucinogens, anabolic steroids, and other regulated chemicals.

The DEA, the Department of Health and Human Services, and the FDA are in charge of regulating the CSA. The DEA is responsible for enforcing the CSA and can prosecute any violators on a domestic and international level. Any individual who handles, stores, orders, or distributes controlled substances must be registered with the DEA and given a DEA number.

The CSA categorizes narcotics into **schedules** based on abuse potential and safety. The schedules range from CI – CV.

- **Schedule I (CI)** are illegal drugs. They are considered not to have any medical value, and they also pose severe safety concerns and have the most abuse potential. Drugs in this class include heroin, LSD, Ecstasy, mescaline, MDMA, GHB, psilocybin, methaqualone, khat, and bath salts. Marijuana is still considered, on a federal level, to be a CI narcotic, although some state laws have changed to allow marijuana to be used for medical and/or recreational use.

- **Schedule II (CII)** are legal drugs with a high potential for abuse. CII drugs do have medical value but are used under severe restrictions. Drugs in this class include opioids, amphetamines, barbiturates, cocaine, and methylphenidate (Ritalin).

- **Schedule III (CIII)** are legal drugs that have the potential for abuse but are less abused and safer than CII narcotics. These drugs have low to moderate potential for physical abuse but high potential for psychological abuse. Drugs in this class include anabolic steroids and low-dose opioids (usually combined with aspirin or acetaminophen [Tylenol]).

- **Schedule IV (CIV)** are legal drugs that have a low potential for physical abuse and a moderate potential for psychological abuse.

**HELPFUL HINT**

When a state controlled-substance law is more stringent than a federal law, the state board of pharmacy will require pharmacies to adhere to the stricter state requirements.

**HELPFUL HINT**

The schedule of the drug is imprinted on the stock bottles of controlled substances. For example, a stock bottle for alprazolam 0.5 mg tablets will have CIV imprinted on it.

Tranquilizers and sleeping medicines are in this schedule. Drugs in this class include benzodiazepines, tramadol, and carisoprodol.

- **Schedule V (CV)** are legal drugs that have a low potential for physical and psychological abuse. Drugs in this class are usually low-dose narcotics or stimulants combined with other medications (e.g., diphenoxylate and atropine [Lonox] and cough medicines with codeine).

## QUICK REVIEW QUESTION

2. Which of the following medications is a Schedule IV drug?

   **A)** cocaine

   **B)** marijuana

   **C)** diazepam

   **D)** hydrocodone

# DEA Registration for Controlled Substances

The DEA enforces the Controlled Substances Act to prevent the diversion and abuse of both controlled substances and chemicals regulated by the FDA. The DEA is involved in every aspect of the handling and distribution of controlled substances and regulated chemicals. They require accurate recordkeeping and compliance from pharmacies, wholesalers, and distributors.

The DEA restricts access to controlled substances and requires all entities that prepare, handle, or distribute controlled substances to fill out an application for **DEA registration**. When the DEA approves registration, it will then give the entity a DEA registration number. Entities that require DEA registration include physicians, drug distributors, drug importers, drug exporters, drug manufacturers, and pharmacies. The application form for DEA registrants is **DEA Form 224**. DEA registration forms are available online at www.deadiversion.usdoj.gov/drugreg.

Once the entity registers with the DEA, it then receives a unique DEA number. The **DEA number** is necessary for the dispensing and distribution of controlled substances. DEA numbers are also used in pharmacy billing; some insurance claims may be denied if the DEA number is incorrect.

Pharmacy technicians must know how to verify a DEA number. A DEA formula can also be calculated to ensure the number is correct.

In the example below, a patient has just dropped off a prescription for a controlled substance. The prescription states that the patient needs morphine IR 30 mg tablets. The physician's name is Dr. May Long, and her DEA number is AL2455562.

To verify that the DEA number is correct, follow this **DEA formula**:

1. A valid DEA number will consist of two letters, six numbers, and one check digit at the end.

2. The first letter of the DEA number is the **DEA registrant** type. Some registrants only have authorization to distribute or manufacture. Other registrants are only allowed to use controlled substances for use in research and labs. Still others, such as practitioners, can write prescriptions for patients. As a pharmacy technician, you will normally encounter DEA numbers that begin with A, B, C, or M. A complete list of registrant types follows.

   A.  deprecated (used by older entities)

   B.  hospital or clinic

   C.  practitioner

   D.  teaching institution

   E.  manufacturer

   F.  distributor

   G.  researcher

   H.  analytical lab

   J.  importer

   K.  exporter

   L.  reverse distributor

   M.  mid-level practitioner

   **P. to U.**  narcotic treatment program

   X.  Suboxone/Subutex prescribing program

3. The second letter is the first letter of the last name of the practitioner. In the example, this would be **L**.

4. To verify the number, the next step is to add the first, third and fifth numbers in the DEA number. In the example, this would be 2 + 5 + 5 = 12.

5. The next step is to add the second, fourth, and sixth number together and multiply by 2. Here, the arithmetic would be 4 + 5 + 6 = 15; 15 × 2 = 30.

6. Finally, the 12 and 30 are added together. The last number should match the last digit in the DEA number. In this example, 12 + 30 = 42. 2 is the last digit in the DEA number: AL2455562.

✓ **CHECK YOUR UNDERSTANDING**

Practice the DEA formula by using these samples: AW3284065, AG4342793, FN5623740, AR5472612, and BN6428521.

## QUICK REVIEW QUESTION

3. Which DEA registrant type is used for a hospital or clinic?

   A) B

   B) M

   C) L

   D) A

## Dispensing of Controlled Substances

### Verifying Patient Information

When the patient drops off a controlled prescription, the pharmacy technician must obtain the information listed below—especially for CII drugs—to be sure the prescription is correctly written by the physician.

- date the prescription was written
- patient's full name and address
- practitioner's name, full address, phone number, and DEA number
- directions for use
- quantity
- number of refills (if allowed)
- manual signature of prescriber

After the technician receives a controlled prescription, the next step is to verify the DEA number as explained above. If there are any discrepancies or questions about the validity of the prescription, or if the DEA number is not verifiable, the pharmacist should be notified. The pharmacist will then take steps, like calling the prescriber, to verify the prescription.

Next, the technician checks the patient's profile. It is essential to look for duplicate drug therapies when dispensing controlled substances. Taking multiple controlled substances can have serious or even fatal consequences. Sometimes a patient may have already been prescribed a medication for another condition or procedure, and not realize the medications are similar. Other times, a patient may have dependency issues; they may be trying to fill multiple prescriptions from different physicians. Any questionable circumstances should always be brought to the attention of the pharmacist.

### QUICK REVIEW QUESTION

4. Which information does NOT need to be checked on a controlled prescription when the patient drops it off?

A) the manual signature of the prescriber

B) the date the prescription was written

C) the patient's full name and address

D) the patient's signature

### Prescription Requirements by Schedule

CII prescriptions must be signed manually in ink by the prescriber. The prescription becomes invalid thirty days after it is written, and the prescriber must submit a new prescription. CII prescriptions can only be written for a thirty-day supply and cannot have refills. The prescriber must write a new prescription for additional fills.

For schedules CIII – CV, the original prescription must be manually signed by the physician. When refilling CIII – CV drugs, the physician can write up to six months of additional refills (the original fill plus five refills), but if the patient needs a refill and none are left on the original prescription, the patient must have a new prescription written by the doctor. It is important to check the date of the last refill on a controlled substance. If the patient is trying to refill the prescription too early, that patient may be abusing the medication and not complying with the directions for use. Oral prescriptions are only allowed in emergencies.

Hard copies of prescriptions must be kept on file in the pharmacy for at least two years. Non-controlled and controlled prescriptions can be filed using one of three separate prescription file systems.

- **Three-file system**: In this system, the pharmacy keeps three files. One file is used exclusively for CII prescriptions, one for CIII – CV prescriptions, and one for non-controlled prescriptions.

- **Two-file system**: In this system one file only contains CII prescriptions and the other contains all other prescriptions. Because the second file contains both controlled and non-controlled medications, the DEA requires identification of the controlled drugs with a red *C* stamp placed on the lower right-hand corner of CIII – CV prescriptions.

- **Alternative two-file system**: With this system all controlled substances are placed in one folder and non-controlled medications in another folder. The CIII – CV prescriptions must still have the *C* stamp in the lower right-hand corner.

## QUICK REVIEW QUESTION

5.  When does a Schedule II prescription become invalid?

   **A)** five days after it is written

   **B)** seven days after it is written

   **C)** thirty days after it is written

   **D)** six months after it is written

## Electronic Prescriptions

Transmitting an **electronic prescription** is called e-prescribing. **E-prescribing** allows pharmacies, nurses, and physicians to communicate and send prescriptions through computer-based transmission and helps provide error-free, accurate prescriptions and information to other health care entities.

Although e-prescribing has many benefits, problems arise with controlled substances. In 2010, the DEA issued new rules on e-prescribing controlled substances, which said CII – CV prescriptions could be transmitted electronically *only if* both the physician and pharmacy software systems were certified to do so by a third-party auditor.

 **HELPFUL HINT**

For more information and updates on electronic prescriptions for controlled substances, visit the DEA's website at www.deadiversion.usdoj.gov/ecomm/e_rx/index.html.

Although it is believed that e-prescribing controlled prescriptions will help prevent medication errors, many pharmacies and physicians' offices still do not have the required software and have not met the DEA requirements for transmitting controlled prescriptions electronically.

## QUICK REVIEW QUESTION

**6.** According to the DEA, what is the main requirement for a pharmacy or physician's office to e-prescribe controlled substances?

   **A)** There must be a manual signature from the physician.

   **B)** The patient must have an ER.

   **C)** The pharmacy and doctor's office must be certified to do so by a third-party auditor.

   **D)** The pharmacy and doctor's office must be authorized by the state BOP.

## Fill Process of Controlled Substances

CII narcotics are stored in a locked narcotics cabinet that can only be accessed by the pharmacist. Depending on state and business-related policies, most pharmacists fill CII narcotics themselves to avoid any counting discrepancies. Pharmacy technicians, however, can fill prescriptions for CIII – CV narcotics. Most pharmacy practices require the pharmacist and technicians to double count and initial the quantity of controlled substances on the label, verifying the medication was counted twice to avoid count discrepancies and inventory issues.

Controlled substances labels have specific requirements under state and federal law. Besides the pharmacy name, address, and phone number, the label must also include the date of fill, prescriber's name, National Drug Code (NDC) number of drug, patient's name, patient's address, order number, directions for use, and any auxiliary labels. Federal guidelines require all controlled substance labels to state, "Caution: Federal law prohibits the transfer of this drug to any person other than the patient for whom it was prescribed."

 **DID YOU KNOW?**

Most prescription pads are tamper-resistant, meaning if an individual attempts to copy a prescription, VOID will show up on the background of the prescription.

## QUICK REVIEW QUESTION

**7.** To verify that a controlled substance medication was counted correctly, the pharmacist and the pharmacy technician must:

   **A)** double count and initial the quantity of the medication.

   **B)** call the prescriber to verify the prescription.

   **C)** store the controlled substance in a locked narcotics cabinet.

   **D)** count the medication in front of the patient.

## Perpetual Inventory

**Perpetual inventory** is required for all CII drugs. Although most inventory in pharmacies is done electronically, perpetual inventory of CII drugs must still be handwritten and signed by a pharmacist when a CII drug has been received into inventory, dispensed to a patient, or the CII drug has been disposed of. Perpetual inventories must be reconciled and verified every ten days to avoid counting discrepancies. CIII – CV drugs may be estimated unless the bulk container contains more than 1,000 units; then it must have an exact count.

On a CII perpetual inventory log, the name of the drug, the item number of the drug, and sheet number are listed on top of the page. The sheet is then divided into three sections that state when the drug is ordered, received, and sold.

- In the *ordered* section, the pharmacist is required to state the date ordered, the order number, the vendor, and the quantity.

- When the order is received, in the *received* section, the pharmacist marks the date received and the quantity. If the drug is backordered, the pharmacist marks the backorder box and/or states the date the vendor is expecting the drug to be available.

- In the *sold* section, the pharmacist writes the date, order number, and the quantity dispensed. After each drug has been entered as ordered, received, and sold, the pharmacist must calculate the quantity balance, sign, and add any necessary comments.

## QUICK REVIEW QUESTION

8.  What is NOT documented on a perpetual inventory log?
    A) CII drug information when ordered from the drug manufacturer
    B) the patient to whom the CII drug was prescribed
    C) CII drugs received by the drug manufacturer
    D) the balance of the quantity for the specific CII drug after each CII drug transaction is recorded

## Emergency Dispensing

The physician may only call in an oral prescription in place of a written one in an emergency and under special circumstances. Emergency dispensing is used when a physician determines that a CII drug is required as soon as possible, and there is no other alternative treatment available for the patient. For example, emergency dispensing may be considered if a patient is in hospice. The pharmacist will then fill the prescription in **good faith**, meaning the pharmacist expects the physician to send a written and signed prescription within seven days or less, depending on state laws.

Other guidelines for emergency dispensing follow.

- Emergency dispensing can be used if a physician is out of the area and cannot give the pharmacist a written prescription.

- The physician must give the pharmacist the patient's name, address, drug name, drug dosage, drug strength, dosage form, route of administration, physician's name, address, phone number, and DEA number. The pharmacist must document the information in writing.

- The quantity dispensed can only be enough to sustain the patient during the emergency time period, which should not exceed three days.
- The pharmacist must document on the prescription that it was dispensed in an emergency.
- The pharmacist must verify the physician's authority.
- After the oral prescription, the physician must submit a hard copy prescription to the pharmacist within seven days with the statement *Authorization for Emergency Dispensing* written on it. If the physician fails to complete these steps, the DEA must be informed.
- The hard copy must be attached to and filed with the oral prescription.
- There might be additional requirements based on the BOP regulation of the state in which the CII drug was dispensed.

With CIII – CV prescriptions, if the pharmacy does not have enough of a drug in stock to fill the full quantity of the prescription, the pharmacist can give the patient a **partial fill** to hold the patient over until the rest of the prescription can be filled. In these cases, the pharmacist may prorate the price of the prescription, and the patient can call in a refill when needed; otherwise, the pharmacy may owe the additional quantity to the patient and, when the drug is available, the patient can pick up the additional quantity at no charge. In this event, the pharmacist must mark on the label the amount of pills given and the amount owed to the patient.

With CII prescriptions, the pharmacist may also partially fill for a patient. If the pharmacist is unable to dispense the remaining quantity within seventy-two hours, the physician must be notified, and the physician must write a new prescription for the additional quantity. Partial fills must be noted on the hard copy of the prescription along with the amount filled.

## QUICK REVIEW QUESTION

9.  Which of the following is NOT a valid reason for dispensing an emergency oral prescription?

    **A)** The patient is terminally ill or in hospice.

    **B)** A Schedule II drug is required as soon as possible.

    **C)** The patient did not refill their medication before it expired.

    **D)** The prescriber determines there's no alternative method of treatment.

## Storage and Security Requirements

All controlled substances are stored in a way that obstructs theft or drug diversion. The higher the class of the controlled substance, the more stringent the storage and security requirements of the drug.

CI substances, although very rarely used, must be securely locked and placed in a cabinet with controlled accessibility. **Controlled accessibility** refers to the use of security features that control access to a certain resource. CI drugs are only used in scientific and clinical studies and research.

CIII – CV drugs must also be stored securely. These drugs are stored in pharmacies, clinical research clinics, and scientific labs. Although the drugs can be placed alongside non-controlled drugs, the health care setting itself is secured through strict regulations to prevent diversion. Regulations can include making the health care setting accessible only to authorized personnel who need keys or passwords to enter the facility.

CII drugs are more strongly secured within the health care setting. As with CI drugs, they are closely monitored and under lock and key in specially constructed safety cabinets. Some ways to prevent theft and ensure the security of the health care setting include:

- electronic alarm systems
- self-closing and automatic locking doors
- key- and/or password-control systems
- allowing authorized personnel only
- using security officers in high-crime areas

**HELPFUL HINT**

The DEA provides more information and updates on storage and security of controlled substances online at www.deadiversion.usdoj.gov/21cfr/cfr/1301/1301_71.html.

## QUICK REVIEW QUESTION

10. Which of the following is NOT a way to control theft and drug diversion?
    A) storing all drugs together in a central location
    B) controlled accessibility via keycards
    C) self-locking doors
    D) electronic alarm systems

## Handling Controlled Substances

### Ordering Controlled Substances

Pharmacists are responsible for ordering CII drugs because only individuals who have a DEA number can order them. CII ordering requires **DEA Form 222**. If the form is filled out incorrectly, the distributor cannot process the order. When filling out DEA Form 222, the pharmacist must include the following specific information.

- company name and address
- order date
- name of drug
- order number of the item (up to ten items per form)
- quantity of packages of the item needed
- package size of the item needed

- purchaser's (pharmacist's) signature
- pharmacist's DEA number

## QUICK REVIEW QUESTION

11. Which is NOT required on DEA Form 222 when a pharmacist is ordering CII drugs?

    **A)** order number

    **B)** number of packages

    **C)** size of package

    **D)** doctor's DEA number

 **HELPFUL HINT**

A pharmacy may distribute a CII drug to another pharmacy or health care setting only under certain conditions. The pharmacy or health care setting must be a DEA registrant, and it must use DEA Form 222 to request the drug.

## Receiving Controlled Substances

Pharmacists are required to receive the CII orders. When the order is received, the pharmacist verifies that the order is complete and logs the order in the perpetual inventory book. CII drug records must be complete, accurate, and be kept for two to five years, depending on the state where the pharmacy is located. CII records are kept separately from all other records.

## QUICK REVIEW QUESTION

12. Once the pharmacy has received an order for a Schedule II medication, the prescription must be verified by the:

    **A)** pharmacy technician.

    **B)** distributor.

    **C)** DEA.

    **D)** pharmacist.

## Expired Controlled Substances

In the course of regular business, pharmacies will have controlled substances in stock that cannot be dispensed to patients. These medications may be expired, damaged, or otherwise unusable (e.g., remaining medication in a single-use vial). The DEA requires that these controlled substances be destroyed so that they are "non-retrievable," meaning they cannot be used or transformed back into a controlled substance.

Most pharmacies use a **reverse distributor** that collects unusable controlled substances and destroys them. The reverse distributor might come to the pharmacy to collect these medications, or the pharmacy might package and ship the medications using DEA Form 222. Reverse distributors must be used for medications that have been dispensed to a patient that the patient returns to the pharmacy or any medications for which the pharmacy needs reimbursement.

In limited cases the pharmacy might choose to destroy controlled substances. When this occurs, the pharmacy must complete **DEA Form 41**. The form must be kept on file for two years but only needs to be submitted to the DEA if requested. Destruction of the drugs must be witnessed by two people. Approved witnesses include pharmacists, nurses, certain other health care practitioners, and law enforcement officers.

---

## QUICK REVIEW QUESTION

**13.** When must Form 41 be submitted to the DEA?

    **A)** immediately

    **B)** within one week

    **C)** within one month

    **D)** when requested

---

## Theft or Loss of Controlled Substances

Any theft or loss of a controlled substance must be documented, and the pharmacist must contact their local DEA office. Significant losses must be reported immediately. For smaller losses or thefts of controlled substances, pharmacists fill out **DEA Form 106**. The form includes the pharmacy's name, address, phone number, DEA number, date of loss or theft, list of items stolen or lost, local police department information, and information about the container and labels with a description and costs. Copies of DEA Form 106 are then sent to the state BOP, the local police, and the DEA.

---

## QUICK REVIEW QUESTION

**14.** Whom should the pharmacist contact first if the theft or loss of a controlled substance occurs?

    **A)** the local police

    **B)** the Drug Enforcement Administration

    **C)** the State Board of Pharmacy

    **D)** the Bureau of Alcohol, Tobacco and Firearms

---

## DEA Inspections

DEA inspections are mandated by the Controlled Substances Act and require administrative search warrants. Before entering a DEA-registered business, the inspectors must state the purpose of the inspection and identify themselves. During consensual inspections, the DEA checks the accuracy of DEA- and state BOP-required controlled substances recordkeeping. DEA inspections are usually performed with a representative of the BOP. The inspectors also check for correct and up-to-date DEA registrants, certifications, and registrations.

Proper controlled substance records make the inspection quick and efficient. Records checked include all invoices and receipts for orders, receiving, distribution, inventory, DEA Form 222s, and the file systems for those CII and CIII – CV prescriptions filled. Records are kept on file for at least two years—sometimes longer depending on state requirements.

**HELPFUL HINT**

When a DEA inspector identifies him- or herself, the pharmacy technician must refer the DEA agent to the pharmacist-in-charge. Otherwise the DEA agent will give the pharmacy a negative mark for noncompliance during the DEA inspection.

In emergencies, dangerous health situations, or if the inspection is of a special state statute category, DEA agents may not have an administrative search warrant but still must identify themselves and their purpose. Pharmacy technicians are required to immediately refer the DEA agent to the pharmacist-in-charge.

## QUICK REVIEW QUESTION

**15.** What must the pharmacy technician immediately do if DEA agents identify themselves for an inspection?

**A)** retrieve all records needed for the inspection

**B)** allow the agents into the pharmacy and start showing them around

**C)** show the inspectors where the file system is located

**D)** refer the agents to the pharmacist-in-charge

## Prescription Monitoring

Many states now participate in **prescription drug monitoring programs (PDMP)**. These programs identify possible abuse and diversion of controlled substances. The statewide electronic database is used by statewide regulatory, administrative, and law enforcement agencies. The DEA is not involved in state monitoring programs. The monitoring programs not only identify discrepancies within a patient's controlled prescription history, but can also find discrepancies with prescribers and pharmacies in the dispensing of controlled drugs. For more information about PDMPs, visit www.pmpalliance.org.

The **National Alliance for Model State Drug Laws (NAMSDL)** states that PDMPs:

- support access to legitimate medical use of controlled substances
- identify and deter or prevent drug abuse and diversion
- facilitate and encourage the identification of, intervention with, and treatment of persons addicted to prescription drugs
- inform public health initiatives by outlining use and abuse trends
- educate individuals about PDMPs and the use of, abuse and diversion of, and addiction to prescription drugs

Some states have begun to participate in nationwide programs that monitor the prescription histories of potential drug abusers across state lines. This program is called **NABP PMP InterConnect**. More than thirty states currently participate in the program.

## QUICK REVIEW QUESTION

**16.** Which is NOT a purpose of the PDMP?

**A)** to track patients with chronic pain and deter them from taking narcotics

**B)** to support access to legitimate medical use of controlled substances

**C)** to identify and deter or prevent drug abuse and diversion

**D)** to inform public health initiatives through outlining use and abuse trends

## Restricted Drug Programs

### Restriction on Sales of Products Containing Ephedrine and Pseudoephedrine

**The Combat Methamphetamine Epidemic Act of 2005 (CMEA)** regulates the over-the-counter sales of **ephedrine** and **pseudoephedrine**, chemicals commonly used in the production of methamphetamine. In retail pharmacy, enforcing the CMEA requirements is an important task of the pharmacy technician.

CMEA is an amendment to the CSA. The act ensures there is a sufficient supply of ephedrine and pseudoephedrine for medical purposes while deterring illegal uses of the drugs. The act requires retailers to place products containing ephedrine and pseudoephedrine out of direct customer access. Customers must purchase these products at the pharmacy counter; employees must ask customers for their photo ID and signature and keep this information in sales logbooks. Furthermore, sellers of ephedrine and pseudoephedrine must obtain self-certification, and employees must receive required training.

Retail customers may buy no more than 3.6 grams of ephedrine or pseudoephedrine products a day. Furthermore, retail customers may buy no more than 9 grams of these products every thirty days (or 7.5 grams by mail order). Prescription drugs are exempt from logbook requirements.

 **HELPFUL HINT**

Mississippi and Oregon require prescriptions for ephedrine and pseudoephedrine.

**CHECK YOUR UNDERSTANDING**

If each Sudafed pill contains 30 mg of pseudoephedrine, how many pills could a patient buy every thirty days if the limit is 9 grams?

### QUICK REVIEW QUESTION

**17.** Which of the following is NOT a requirement of the CMEA?

**A)** A thirty-day supply of medication containing ephedrine or pseudoephedrine is limited to 9 grams in retail environments.

**B)** Sellers must obtain self-certification.

**C)** Patients are required to have a prescription to receive ephedrine and pseudoephedrine.

**D)** Selling products containing ephedrine or pseudoephedrine requires employee training.

### Risk Evaluation and Mitigation Strategies

When a drug has adverse effects that may outweighs the therapeutic benefits, the FDA will require a manufacturer to develop a **Risk Evaluation and Mitigation Strategy (REMS)**. The purpose of the REMS is to decrease the occurrence and severity of a drug's possible serious adverse effects. There are different types of REMS, but most include communication literature and protocols for health care providers. Information about the drug's risks are outlined in **packaged inserts**, which are given to everyone involved, including patients, health care providers, and the pharmacy.

A pharmacy that dispenses medications with a REMS must dispense those medications according to the requirements of the REMS. Pharmacists and sometimes technicians may require additional training according to the specification of a REMS. For example, clozapine has a REMS because it may lead to neutropenia (low white-blood cell count). To dispense clozapine, the pharmacy must be certified, and staff must obtain a **Predispense Authorization** from the clozapine REMS program for each patient.

## QUICK REVIEW QUESTION

**18.** Risk Evaluation and Mitigation Strategies (REMS) are regulated and enforced by the:

**A)** FDA.

**B)** DEA.

**C)** drug manufacturer.

**D)** prescribing provider.

## Drug Recalls

Sometimes a manufacturer will issue a **recall** of a particular drug batch because the product has been determined to be harmful. Reasons for a recall include defective products, contamination, incorrect labelling, FDA interference, or improper production.

In these cases, the manufacturer will send **recall notices** to the pharmacy. The pharmacy must act on these immediately to prevent the consumer from receiving the recalled drug. Notices will provide specific information about the product, including the drug name, lot number, and the reason for the recall.

Pharmacies have specific policies and procedures in place to ensure that the recalled drug is pulled from the shelves, documented, and returned based on recall procedures. This includes notifying the manufacturer and the FDA of compliance with the removal of the recalled drug.

Recalled medications should be removed from inventory and placed in a designated area until they are returned or disposed of as required by the recall notice. Technicians must check all inventory, including the shelving in the pharmacy as well as the med units and automated drug dispensing systems located in the institutional pharmacy. If the recalled product is not in stock, the pharmacy must still send the recall form back to the FDA and manufacturer stating this fact.

The pharmacy is also required to contact affected patients if the pharmacy dispensed the recalled product. In these cases, the pharmacy or doctor's office may contact the patient to check the lot number of the dispensed medication. If the patient received a recalled product, the patient is asked to return the medication for a replacement. The pharmacy then must contact the manufacturer for replacement of the drug.

 **HELPFUL HINT**

Lot numbers are crucial to the recall because they identify the defective batch of the drug.

 **HELPFUL HINT**

A current listing of drug recalls is available online at www.fda.gov/Drugs/Drugsafety/DrugRecalls.

There are three levels of recalls. They can be conducted by the FDA or the manufacturer. The levels are determined by the urgency and severity of the recall.

- **Class I recall**: There is a probability that use of or exposure to the product could cause an adverse event, health consequences, or death.

- **Class II recall**: The product may cause temporary health problems, and there is a remote probability of an adverse health event.

- **Class III recall**: The product is not likely to cause an adverse event but has violated FDA regulations.

**FDA market withdrawals** can happen when a product has a minor violation that does not require legal action, but the product still must be removed from the market to correct the violation.

## QUICK REVIEW QUESTION

**19.** A Class II recall occurs when:

**A)** the product is not likely to cause an adverse event but has violated FDA regulations.

**B)** a product has a minor violation that does not require legal action, but the product still must be removed from the market to correct the violation.

**C)** the product may cause temporary health problems, and there is a remote probability of an adverse health event.

**D)** there is a probability that the use of or exposure to the product could cause an adverse event, health consequences, or death.

1.  **B)** The Drug Enforcement Agency (DEA) is responsible for monitoring the handling and distribution of controlled substances.

2.  **C)** Benzodiazepines, including diazepam, are classified as Schedule IV drugs.

3.  **A)** *B* is used for a hospital or clinic.

4.  **D)** The patient's signature is not required on a controlled prescription.

5.  **B)** Schedule II prescriptions must be filled within seven days, or the patient will need a new prescription.

6.  **C)** The entities (both pharmacy and doctor's office) must be certified and audited by a third-party auditor to be able to e-prescribe controlled substances.

7.  **A)** In most pharmacies, the pharmacist and the pharmacy technician must double count and initial the label of controlled substance medications.

8.  **B)** Patient names are not listed on the perpetual inventory log.

9.  **C)** An expired prescription is not a valid reason to dispense an emergency prescription.

10. **A)** To prevent theft and diversion, controlled substances should be stored separately from other drugs. Schedule II drugs must be kept in a locked safety cabinet where they are accessible only by key or password.

11. **D)** The purchaser's (pharmacist's) DEA number is required, not the doctor's.

12. **D)** The pharmacist must verify all prescriptions for Schedule II drugs.

13. **D)** Form 41 only needs to be submitted when requested.

14. **B)** The pharmacist should immediately contact the DEA before anyone else.

15. **D)** Pharmacy technicians should immediately refer the inspectors to the pharmacist-in-charge.

16. **A)** PDMP is not used to track patients who have chronic pain and deter them from taking narcotics.

17. **C)** Patients do not need a prescription to purchase products containing ephedrine or pseudoephedrine in most states.

18. **A)** The FDA can require manufacturers to develop a REMS and may take action against participants who do not adhere to the REMS.

19. **C)** A Class II recall occurs when the product may cause temporary health problems, and there is a remote probability of an adverse health event.

# 3 Patient Safety and Quality Assurance

## Medication Errors

A **medication error** is any health care action or decision that causes an unintended consequence. Each year, nearly 1.5 million medication errors occur in the United States. In pharmacies, it is estimated that nearly 2 percent of all written prescriptions contain some form of medication error. Pharmacy technicians should be familiar with the most common errors that occur in pharmacies.

- **Abnormal doses** occur when the prescribed dose and/or frequency is not consistent with the manufacturer's dosing recommendation. The abnormal dose can result in over/underdose, leading to adverse reactions or a failure in treatment. The pharmacist must be alerted to abnormal doses so the prescriber can correct it.

- **Early refills**—when a patient requests the pharmacy refill a medication before it is due to be refilled—may indicate the patient is taking the medication incorrectly. The pharmacist should be alerted to early refills so they can consult with the patient. If a physician changes a prescription in the middle of a patient's therapy without informing the pharmacy, the pharmacy will need to contact the patient's third-party payer and refill the medication with the updated instructions.

- Patients may be dispensed an **incorrect quantity** of a medication due to counting or clerical errors (e.g., misreading a prescription).

- Medications may be dispensed to the **incorrect patient** if all the patient's information has not been correctly collected and verified.

- The **incorrect drug** may be dispensed due to technician error. This error is more likely to occur with drugs that have similar names or that are shelved close together.

- **Drug preparation errors** occur when the drug is not prepared as prescribed. Technicians must be especially aware of this type of error during compounding.

- A **deteriorated drug error** occurs when an expired drug is used, or the chemical or physical potency and integrity of the drug has been compromised (e.g., it has not been stored properly).
- A **compliance error** occurs when a patient does not take the medication as directed.

## QUICK REVIEW QUESTION

1. A patient was dispensed a thirty-day supply of a medication and has requested a refill after fifteen days. The pharmacy technician should:

   A) fill the prescription as requested.

   B) tell the patient that the prescription cannot be refilled early.

   C) alert the pharmacist.

   D) call the patient's insurance provider.

## Error Prevention

### Look-Alike/Sound-Alike Drug Names

**Look-alike/sound-alike medications** (LASA or SALAD medications) are increasingly a problem for health care professionals. There are a large number of brand and generic drugs available and in development, and some drug names sound or are spelled similarly. These similarities can cause health care professionals to mistakenly dispense or administer the wrong drug.

Some contributing factors to misreading LASA drugs include similar packaging, interruptions while preparing the drug, bad lighting, and incorrect placement of the stock bottles on the shelf. To resolve these factors and avoid confusion, the FDA and the Joint Commission developed the following strategies and requirements:

- Tall Man lettering should be used on labels. When drugs have similar names, they are differentiated by capitalizing the dissimilar letters (e.g., ClomiPHENE and ClomiPRAMINE).

- The Joint Commission requires all LASA medications, along with chemicals and reagents that can be mistaken for drugs, be kept away from other products.

- The Joint Commission also requires that a written policy be displayed in the health care setting specifying necessary precautions and procedures when ordering LASA drugs.

- Health care facilities must define which drugs and products used in the facility qualify as high-risk and develop policies and procedures for the drug or product throughout the dispensing process.

- Finally, health care settings must identify and produce an annual review of all LASA drugs used in the facility.

## TABLE 3.1. Look-Alike/Sound-Alike Drugs

| FDA LIST OF GENERIC LASA DRUGS (FULL) | ISMP LIST OF LASA DRUGS (MOST COMMON) |
|---|---|
| acetaZOLAMIDE/acetoHEXAMIDE | ALPRAZolam/LORazepam/clonazePAM |
| buPROPion/busPIRone | aMILoride/amLODIPine |
| chlorproMAZINE/chlorproPAMIDE | amiVUDine/lamoTRIgine |
| clomiPHENE/clomiPRAMINE | AVINza/INVanz |
| cycloSERINE/cycloSPORINE | carBAMazepine/OXcarbazepine |
| DAUNOrubicin/DOXOrubicin | CeleBREX/CeleXA |
| dimenhyDRINATE/diphenhydrAMINE | clonazePAM/cloNIDine/cloZAPine/cloBAZam/KlonoPIN |
| DOBUTamine/DOPamine | DEPO-Medrol/SOLU-Medrol |
| glipiZIDE/glyBURIDE | diazePAM/dilTIAZem |
| hydrALAZINE/hydrOXYzine/HYDROmorphone | DULoxetine/FLUoxetine/PARoxetine |
| | ePHEDrine/EPINEPHrine |
| medroxyPROGESTERone/methylPREDNISolone/methylTESTOSTERone | fentaNYL/SUFentanil |
| | guaiFENesin/guanFACINE |
| niCARdipine/NIFEdipine | HumaLOG/HumuLIN |
| prednisoLONE/predniSONE | LaMICtal/LamISIL |
| risperiDONE/rOPINIRole | levETIRAcetam/levOCARNitine/levoFLOXacin |
| sulfADIAZINE/sulfiSOXAZOLE | metFORMIN/metroNIDAZOLE |
| TOLAZamide/TOLBUTamide | NexAVAR/NexIUM |
| vinBLAStine/vinCRIStine | NovoLIN/NovoLOG |
| | OLANZapine/QUEtiapine |
| | oxyCODONE/HYDROcodone/OxyCONTIN/oxyMORphone |
| | penicillAMINE/penicillin |
| | PriLOSEC/PROzac |
| | raNITIdine/riMANTAdine |
| | sAXagliptin/SITagliptin/SUMAtriptan |
| | SEROquel/SINEquan |
| | TEGretol/TRENtal |
| | tiaGABine/tiZANidine |
| | traMADol/traZODone |
| | valACYclovir/valGANciclovir |
| | ZyPREXA/ZyrTEC |

Pharmacy staff can be proactive in preventing LASA errors by doing the following:

- Pharmacy staff must not store LASA drugs alphabetically with other drug products; they should place LASA drugs on a separate shelf or in another area of the pharmacy.

- Pharmacy staff must undergo training on the precautions taken with LASA drugs to avoid prescribing errors.

- Pharmacy staff should change the appearance of LASA drugs by using techniques such as bold typing, color codes, highlighting, circling, or Tall Man lettering to emphasize dissimilar parts of the drug name. The same method must be used throughout the chosen medication management system, including the computer system, medication administration records (MARs), and in nursing unit med rooms and bins.

- Pharmacy staff must apply auxiliary labels that warn about LASA drugs.
- Pharmacy staff must avoid abbreviations when entering, filling, or dispensing LASA drugs.
- Pharmacy staff must add a prompt in the pharmacy computer system that warns when LASA drugs are dispensed.

## QUICK REVIEW QUESTION

2. Which of the following strategies is used to prevent look-alike/sound-alike (LASA) medication errors?

    **A)** placing LASA medications in similar packaging

    **B)** using Tall Man lettering

    **C)** using abbreviations

    **D)** storing all LASA medications on the same shelf

## Abbreviation Errors

Although using abbreviations in the pharmacy saves time and improves efficiency, **abbreviation errors** can also result in misinterpretations, especially if two abbreviations are similar. The Joint Commission has created an official *Do Not Use* list of abbreviations that can cause medication errors, which applies to all orders and all medication-related documentation that is handwritten (including free-text computer entry) or on pre-printed forms.

### TABLE 3.2. Official *Do Not Use* Abbreviation List

| DO NOT USE | POTENTIAL PROBLEM | USE INSTEAD |
|---|---|---|
| U, u (unit) | Mistaken for *0* (zero), the number *4* (four), or *cc* | Write *unit* |
| IU (international unit) | Mistaken for *IV* (intravenous) or the number *10* (ten) | Write *international unit* |
| Q.D., QD, q.d., qd (daily)<br>Q.O.D., QOD, q.o.d, qod (every other day) | Mistaken for each other<br>Period after the *Q* mistaken for *I* and the *O* mistaken for *I* | Write *daily*<br>Write *every other day* |
| Trailing zero (X.0 mg)*<br>Lack of leading zero (.X mg) | Decimal point is missed | Write *X mg*<br>Write *0.X mg* |
| MS<br>MSO$_4$ and MgSO$_4$ | Can mean morphine sulfate or magnesium sulfate<br>Confused for one another | Write *morphine sulfate*<br>Write *magnesium sulfate* |

*Exception: A trailing zero may be used only where required to demonstrate the level of precision of the value being reported, such as for laboratory results, imaging studies that report size of lesions, or catheter tube sizes. It may not be used in medication orders or other medication-related documentation.

## TABLE 3.3. Additional Abbreviations, Acronyms, and Symbols*

| DO NOT USE | POTENTIAL PROBLEM | USE INSTEAD |
|---|---|---|
| > (greater than) <br> < (less than) | Misinterpreted as the number 7 (seven) or the letter L <br> Confused for one another | Write *greater than* <br> Write *less than* |
| Abbreviations for drug names | Misinterpreted due to similar abbreviations for multiple drugs | Write drug names in full |
| Apothecary units | Unfamiliar to many practitioners <br> Confused with metric units | Use metric units |
| @ | Mistaken for the number 2 (two) | Write *at* |
| cc | Mistaken for *U* (units) when poorly written | Write *mL, ml*, or *milliliters* (*mL* is preferred) |
| µg | Mistaken for *mg* (milligrams) | Write *mcg* or *micrograms* |
| *For POSSIBLE future inclusion in the *Do Not Use* Abbreviation List | | |

## QUICK REVIEW QUESTION

3.   Which of the following dosages is written incorrectly?

   **A)**   10 mg

   **B)**   1 mg

   **C)**   0.1 mg

   **D)**   1.0 mg

## Check Systems

Preventing medication errors is one of the pharmacist's highest priorities. Pharmacy technicians play a crucial role in preventing errors by assisting the pharmacist with routine tasks so the pharmacist can focus on verification of prescription orders. Pharmacy technicians also help the pharmacist by being vigilant and checking their work through **multiple check systems**.

The first check system is at **prescription drop-off**. Technicians stationed at the drop-off window work with the patient. They create a checklist of important information needed to accurately enter the prescription and alert the pharmacist to any issues requiring the pharmacist's attention.

During order entry, technicians who enter the prescription information into the pharmacy software system use their knowledge of pharmacy terminology and drug names to prevent medication errors and enhance patient safety. **Computerization** and **automation** also help technicians by increasing accuracy and decreasing errors, but these are only tools. Technicians are alerted to possible warnings that include interaction, allergies, and duplications. Technicians must work with the pharmacist to decide if the warning can be overridden or if the provider must intervene.

Depending on the pharmacy's policies and procedures, some technicians may be allowed to carry out certain overrides—for instance, if a patient is going on vacation and needs an early refill. If the technician gets an authorization code from the third-party payer allowing the early refill, the pharmacy's policies and procedures may allow the technician to override the prescription.

During the **dispensing process**, another check system, medication errors can occur in a few ways. First, it is important for the fill technician to check the hard copy against the prescription label that was generated by the order entry technician. This way, the fill technician is double checking the order entry technician's work for errors and possibly preventing a dispensing error.

Another error can happen if the fill technician incorrectly reads the label: one consequence could be choosing the incorrect LASA drug from the shelf, for example. Furthermore, a technician could be rushed and choose the correct drug but not the correct strength. In these cases, it is crucial to check the National Drug Code (NDC) number and the illustration on the label. Tools like barcode technology and vial-filling systems that count out the amount of pills needed when the label is generated can help the technician prevent errors.

The next check system is the **pharmacist verification process**. The pharmacist thoroughly checks the prescription order from order entry through the dispensing process. Through scanning and barcode technology, the pharmacy software system will alert the pharmacist to any issues that require reconciliation. The pharmacist will then check the NDC number with the stock bottle, check the labeling for accuracy, and make sure the drug is correct by verifying the illustration image.

The last check system—**point of sale**—is at the check-out counter. Prevention of errors at this stage includes using a second identifier in addition to the name at the point of sale. The technician will ask the patient for an address, phone number, or date of birth. This ensures that the medication was filled for the correct patient, especially if the prescription was called in or sent electronically to the pharmacy.

Verifying the quantity of prescriptions for pickup is important, too. Many patients pick up more than one prescription at a time; failure to distribute all their medications at once is poor customer service. Sometimes a medication may be overlooked or not yet filled. In these cases, the technician should check the patient's profile in the computer system to determine the problem. For example, the pharmacist may be waiting for the patient's doctor to call in a new prescription, or the patient may have called in a refill too soon.

Furthermore, pharmacies have systems to refer patients to the pharmacist for high-risk medications or alert them to changes in medication dosages or strengths. Some pharmacies place notes on the bag or use other internal protocols directing technicians to refer patients to a pharmacist for counseling.

4. A pharmacy technician incorrectly reads a label and prepares a prescription for warfarin 5 mg instead of warfarin 2.5 mg. Which of the following multiple-check systems has failed?

   **A)** data entry

   **B)** verification

   **C)** drop-off

   **D)** dispensing

## High-Alert Medications

In institutional settings, **high-alert medications** may cause significant harm to a patient if they are used in error. Although the drugs are not consistently prescribed wrong, when they are, the results can be much more devastating for the patient. There are no legal requirements for pharmacies to meet when dispensing high-alert medications. However, most institutions will have protocols in place to ensure that these medications are dispensed with no errors. High-alert medications include:

- heparin
- opioids
- potassium chloride injections
- insulin
- chemotherapeutic agents
- neuromuscular blocking agents

## QUICK REVIEW QUESTION

5. Which of the following medications is NOT a high-alert medication?

   **A)** neuromuscular blocking agents

   **B)** heparin

   **C)** insulin

   **D)** penicillin

## What to Do if an Error Occurs

### Error Reporting

Whenever the technician commits or discovers a medication error, they must inform their supervisor immediately. Failure to inform supervisors of an error can be grounds for dismissal.

To help prevent future medication errors, technicians should also report errors to either the FDA's **MedWatch** program or the ISMP **National Medication Errors Reporting Program**. Both programs help the FDA, manufacturers, and pharmacy professionals implement protocols to prevent recurring errors. MedWatch is a voluntary FDA program that offers a channel to anonymously report medication errors and adverse effects. The ISMP is a nonprofit that focuses on collecting and reporting on medication errors.

Reports on medication errors can be filed online for both programs. When reporting the error, the technician should include:

- an explanation of what went wrong, the contributing factors, and how the error was discovered

- the name(s) of the medication, the form, dosage strength, and manufacturer's name

- supplemental information like pictures or labels

Sometimes, a medication error *almost* happens but ultimately does not. These events are called **near-misses**. Even though the error did not occur (and thus no patients were harmed), it is still considered an error and should be reported similarly.

**HELPFUL HINT**

Although pharmacy technicians cannot counsel a patient who may have experienced a medication error, they can encourage patients to consult with the pharmacist.

---

## QUICK REVIEW QUESTION

6. A patient who has picked up a medication returns the next day and tells the technician that they received the wrong medication. They state that they didn't take any of the medication. The technician should:

    **A)** immediately inform the pharmacist of the error.

    **B)** file a near-miss report.

    **C)** dispense the patient's correct prescription.

    **D)** try to find out why the patient received the wrong medication.

---

## Error Analysis

If an error does occur, it is important to focus on its cause and how to improve the work habits that contributed to the problem. By using systemic reviews to identify common factors that lead to errors, pharmacies can develop and implement strategies that improve the quality of pharmacy workflow while limiting mistakes. This process is referred to as **continuous quality improvement (CQI)**.

**Failure mode and effects analysis (FMEA)** is an ongoing quality multidisciplinary improvement process carried out by health care organizations. FMEA helps pharmacies inspect new products and services to determine points of possible failure and the effects of the failure before any error can actually happen. FMEA is a proactive process that determines steps that can be taken to avoid errors before the product or service is purchased. For example, to reduce medication errors, a multidisciplinary team will use FMEA to assess new drugs before considering placement of the drug in the health care organization's formulary. To complete the process, a series of steps must be taken.

- **Step One**: The multidisciplinary team first determines how the product is to be used. This will be deliberated thoroughly, from purchasing to administering the drug. Questions that would be considered include: What type of patient needs the drug? Who would prescribe the drug? How is the drug stored? How is the drug prepared and administered?

- **Step Two**: While discussing how the drug is used, the team then examines possible failures of the drug, including whether the labeling of the drug could be mistaken for another similarly packaged drug, if the drug could be mistaken for another drug, or if errors could occur during the administration of the drug.

- **Step Three**: After identifying any failures in the process, the team then determines the likelihood and consequences of the mistake. What adverse events could happen if the patient receives the drug at the wrong time, dose, route of administration, or rate?

- **Step Four**: The team factors in any of the patient's pre-existing conditions and any processes already in place that may cause an error before the drug reaches the patient. Then, team members use their individual, specialized knowledge to account for human factors to determine the effectiveness of the drug.

- **Step Five**: If any significant errors occur during the evaluation, the team takes actions to detect, prevent, or minimize the consequences. Some examples include using a different product, requiring dosing and concentration methods, using warning systems such as auxiliary labels or computer alerts, requiring specific drug preparations in the pharmacy, and requiring specific data in the software systems before processing orders.

Methodologies such as FMEA and **root cause analysis (RCA)** can also improve quality and reduce errors in the pharmacy. RCA helps identify the cause of an error after the error occurs. When initiating a CQI project, the **FOCUS-PDCA** cycle can be used as well.

FOCUS stands for:

- **Find** the improvement opportunity.
- **Organize** a group to help in the improvement process.
- **Clarify** current knowledge of the process.
- **Understand** the cause and effect in the process.
- **Select** which improvement needs to take place.

PDCA stands for:

- **Plan** the action needed to solve the problem.
- **Do** the action needed to solve the problem.
- **Check** to be sure the action works properly by studying the results.
- **Act** on the action: proceed with implementing the solution.

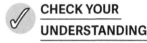

### CHECK YOUR UNDERSTANDING

Despite safeguards to avoid confusion among LASA drugs, a technician entered the wrong drug. The pharmacist catches the mistake during the verification process. What can the technician do in the future to avoid making the same mistake again?

---

## QUICK REVIEW QUESTION

**7.** The goal of root cause analysis is to:

**A)** punish employees who incorrectly dispense medication.

**B)** identify adverse drug effects.

**C)** prevent future medication errors.

**D)** improve customer satisfaction.

---

## Pharmacist Intervention

Technicians are NOT allowed to counsel patients about issues related to pharmacology (e.g., adverse drug reactions, drug interactions, etc.). When patients need such information, technicians must legally (mandated by the OBRA-90 law) offer patients the opportunity to receive **consultation** from the pharmacist on duty. Consultation allows the pharmacist to provide accurate information to the patient and address any concerns the patient may have.

Most state boards of pharmacy require pharmacists to provide consultation only to patients receiving new prescriptions. The pharmacist ensures that the patient understands what type of drug they are prescribed and how to administer the medication properly. For refills, the technicians may only need to ask patients if they have any questions; if they answer yes, they should be directed to the pharmacist for consultation.

The pharmacist should also be consulted when patients have questions about **over the counter (OTC) medications** (drugs that can be purchased without a prescription). Pharmacists can recommend drugs, discuss appropriate dosages, and caution patients about possible interactions and adverse reactions.

Pharmacists may also intervene to educate a patient based on system alerts or warning messages. The pharmacy's computer will run a **drug utilization review (DUR)** on each prescription to identify any possible issues. The result from a DUR is categorized as mild, moderate, or severe, and the pharmacist must use their judgment to assess how to handle each alert. Possible reasons for DUR alerts include:

- drug-drug interactions
- therapeutic duplications
- incorrect dosages
- adverse drug reactions
- allergies
- drug-disease interactions
- special circumstances for administration
- contraindications for pregnancy

**DID YOU KNOW?**

The FMEA helps identify trends in potential errors with drug products and services based on past use experience and informational media tools, such as the ISMP Medication Safety Alert! newsletters. The newsletters can be viewed at www.ismp.org/newsletters/.

**HELPFUL HINT**

Most OTC medications that treat the common cold are not safe for patients with high blood pressure.

### QUICK REVIEW QUESTION

**8.** A patient is picking up a refill for an albuterol inhaler. Which of the following patient questions must be answered by the pharmacist?

    **A)** "Is a spacer included with the prescription?"

    **B)** "How many doses can I take in one day?"

    **C)** "Will my insurance cover the name brand version of this drug?"

    **D)** "How many refills do I have left?"

# Hygiene and Cleaning

## Asepsis

**Asepsis** is the absence of infectious organisms, and **medical asepsis** is the practice of destroying infectious agents outside the body to prevent the spread of disease. Medical asepsis is different from **clean technique**, which also aims to minimize the spread of infectious agents but does not require sterilization. Wearing gloves is an example of clean technique; the gloves are not sterile, but they provide a barrier that prevents the spread of infection.

The most important tool used for medical asepsis is handwashing. **Aseptic handwashing** is a specific technique intended to remove all infectious agents from the hands and wrists.

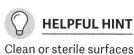

**HELPFUL HINT**

Clean or sterile surfaces become contaminated when they come in contact with pathogens.

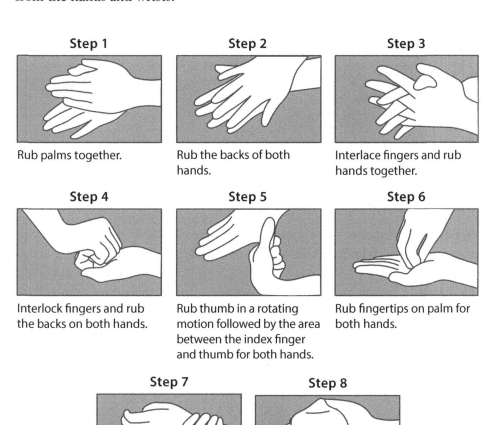

| Step 1 | Step 2 | Step 3 |
|---|---|---|
| Rub palms together. | Rub the backs of both hands. | Interlace fingers and rub hands together. |

| Step 4 | Step 5 | Step 6 |
|---|---|---|
| Interlock fingers and rub the backs on both hands. | Rub thumb in a rotating motion followed by the area between the index finger and thumb for both hands. | Rub fingertips on palm for both hands. |

| Step 7 | Step 8 |
|---|---|
| Rub both wrists in a rotating motion. | Rinse and dry thoroughly. |

*Figure 3.1. Aseptic Handwashing*

Medical asepsis also includes the removal of infectious agents from equipment and other surfaces. This process has three levels.

- Cleaning removes dirt and some infectious agents.

- **Disinfection** kills all pathogens except bacterial spores. Most surfaces in health care settings are disinfected using chemical agents, such as alcohol or chlorine bleach.

- **Sterilization** kills all infectious agents, including bacterial spores. Medical equipment is sterilized using heat or chemicals (e.g., ethylene oxide).

Pharmacy surfaces, including equipment, carts, and shelves, must be disinfected regularly. First, obvious soiling or visible dirt should be removed (usually with soap and water). The surface can then be disinfected with a germicide, usually 70% isopropyl alcohol (IPA). Paper towels, sponges, or mops can be used to clean, but they must be made of a non-shedding material. The schedule for cleaning surfaces is guided by the minimum frequency table displayed in USP 797.

## QUICK REVIEW QUESTION

9. A surface is disinfected after it has been:
    A) cleaned with chlorine bleach.
    B) washed with soap and water.
    C) covered with a drape sheet.
    D) allowed to sit unused for 24 hours.

## Personal Protective Equipment

In addition to handwashing, equipment can be used to prevent the spread of infection. **Personal protective equipment (PPE)** is any item necessary for the prevention of microorganism transmission. PPE includes gloves, gowns, goggles, eye shields, shoe covers, and masks. In the pharmacy, PPE should be used:

- in all sterile environments
- when handling hazardous materials
- during routine cleaning
- during possible exposure to blood-borne pathogens
- around toxic spills

**HELPFUL HINT**

USP 800 lays out the specific items that must be worn when working with hazardous materials, including chemotherapy drugs and other types of compounded sterile products.

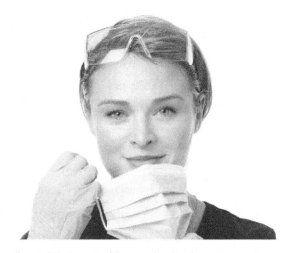

*Figure 3.2. Personal Protective Equipment*

## QUICK REVIEW QUESTION

**10.** The pharmacy technician must wear PPE when:

**A)** stocking inventory in a non-compounding area.

**B)** compounding sterile products.

**C)** handling cash from customers.

**D)** dispensing controlled substances.

1. **C)** The pharmacist should be alerted to early refill requests.

2. **B)** Tall Man lettering helps differentiate LASA medications from each other.

3. **D)** To help avoid medication errors, trailing zeroes (the zero after the decimal point) should not be used.

4. **D)** Pharmacy technicians may incorrectly read the prescription label during the dispensing process when selecting the drug.

5. **D)** Penicillin is not a high-alert medication.

6. **A)** All medication errors should be immediately reported to the pharmacist.

7. **C)** Root cause analysis is performed to identify how an error occurred so that it can be prevented from occurring again in the future.

8. **B)** Questions about drug administration should be directed to the pharmacist.

9. **A)** Chlorine bleach is a disinfectant that will kill most pathogens.

10. **B)** Compounding sterile products requires the use of PPE, including gloves and masks.

# 4 Order Entry and Processing

## Pharmacy Math

### Measurement Systems

The numeric systems used in pharmacy include the metric (or SI), American, and household systems. **Conversion factors** are used to convert measurements in one system into another system.

| TABLE 4.1. Units and Conversion Factors | | |
|---|---|---|
| **DIMENSION** | **AMERICAN** | **METRIC (SI)** |
| length | inch/foot/yard/mile | meter |
| mass | ounce/pound/ton | gram |
| volume | cup/pint/quart/gallon | liter |
| temperature | Fahrenheit | Kelvin/Celsius |

**Conversion Factors**

1 in = 2.54 cm

1 yd = 0.914 m

1 mi = 1.61 km

1 gal = 3.785 L

1 oz = 28.35 g

$°C = \frac{5}{9}(°F - 32)$

$1 \text{ cm}^3 = 1 \text{ mL}$

1 hr = 3600 s

CONTINUE

**HELPFUL HINT**

Metric prefixes are used to write very large or very small numbers. Common prefixes include:

kilo (k): × 1000

centi (c): × 0.01

milli (m): × 0.001

micro (μ): × 0.0000001

| TABLE 4.2. Household System Units and Conversion Factors | |
| --- | --- |
| **HOUSEHOLD UNITS** | **CONVERSION FACTORS** |
| **VOLUME** | |
| teaspoon (tsp or t) | 1 tsp = 5 mL |
| tablespoon (tbsp or T) | 1 tbsp = 3 tsp = 15 mL |
| fluid ounce (fl oz) | 1 fl oz = 30 mL |
| cup (c) | 1 c = 8 fl oz = 240 mL |
| pint (pt) | 1 pt = 2 c = 480 mL |
| quart (qt) | 1 qt = 2 pt = 960 mL |
| gallon (gal) | 1 gal = 4 qt = 3840 mL |
| **WEIGHT** | |
| ounce (oz) | 1 oz = 30 g |
| pound (lb) | 1 lb = 16 oz = 454 g |

**HELPFUL HINT**

When providing instructions to patients in household units, caution them to use a standardized measuring instrument (often provided with the medication).

Pharmacy technicians should also be able to read and manipulate **Roman numerals**. The roman numeral system uses letters to represent numerical values, as shown in Table 4.3.

| TABLE 4.3. Roman Numerals | |
| --- | --- |
| **ROMAN NUMERAL** | **NUMERIC VALUE** |
| I | 1 |
| V | 5 |
| X | 10 |
| L | 50 |
| C | 100 |
| D | 500 |
| M | 1000 |

Numerals are always arranged from greatest to least in value starting with the largest possible number. For example, the number 157 would be written as: 100 + 50 + 5 + 1 + 1 = CLVII.

To avoid adding four of the same numerals in a row, subtraction is used. If a numeral with a smaller value is placed before a numeral with a larger value, the smaller number is subtracted from the bigger number. For example, the number 9 is written as IX (10 − 1 = 9).

## QUICK REVIEW QUESTIONS

1. Convert 3 tablespoons to milliliters.

   **A)** 5 ml

   **B)** 30 ml

   **C)** 45 ml

   **D)** 60 ml

2. Convert 4 ounces to grams.

   **A)** 0.25 g

   **B)** 7.5 g

   **C)** 120 g

   **D)** 240 g

## Ratio, Proportions, and Percentage

A **ratio** describes how many of one thing exists in relation to the number of another thing. For example, if a bag contains 3 apples and 4 oranges, the ratio of apples to oranges is 3 to 4. Ratios can be written using words (3 to 4), fractions ($\frac{3}{4}$), or colons (3:4).

A **proportion** is an equation which states that 2 ratios are equal. Proportions are usually written as 2 fractions joined by an equal sign ($\frac{a}{b} = \frac{c}{d}$), but they can also be written using colons (a : b :: c : d). Note that in a proportion, the units must be the same in both numerators and in both denominators.

A missing value in a proportion can be found by **cross-multiplying**: multiply the numerator of each fraction by the denominator of the other to get an equation with no fractions as shown below. You can then solve the equation using basic algebra.

$$\frac{a}{b} = \frac{c}{d} \rightarrow ad = bc$$

A **percent** describes a part of one hundred. For example, 25 percent means 25 out of 100. A percent is found by dividing the part by the whole:

$$\text{percent} = \frac{\text{part}}{\text{whole}}$$

$$\text{part} = \text{whole} \times \text{percent}$$

For example, if a person has read 5 pages (the part) of a 10-page article (the whole), they've read $\frac{5}{10}$ = 0.5 or 50%. (The percent sign [%] is used once the decimal has been multiplied by 100.)

## QUICK REVIEW QUESTION

3. Grant needs to score 75% on an exam. If the exam has 48 questions, how many does he need to answer correctly?

   **A)** 14

   **B)** 34

   **C)** 36

   **D)** 38

## Specific Gravity

**Specific gravity** is the ratio of the weight of the compound to the weight of the same amount of water (i.e., how heavy a substance is compared to water). For instance, the specific gravity of ethanol is 0.787 g/mL, meaning that ethanol is about 21 percent lighter than water.

When converting between weight and volume it is useful to know a particular compound's specific gravity. The equation for finding the specific gravity of a substance follows:

$$\text{specific gravity} = \frac{\text{weight (g)}}{\text{volume (mL)}}$$

## QUICK REVIEW QUESTION

4. In a compound, the weight of a solid is 45 grams and the volume of the solution used to dissolve it is 500mL. What is the compound's specific gravity?

   **A)** 0.05 g/mL

   **B)** 0.09 g/mL

   **C)** 11.1 g/mL

   **D)** 12.5 g/mL

## Concentrations

**Concentration** refers to the amount of a particular substance in a given volume, or the substance's strength. The more of a substance that is in a given volume, the higher the concentration of the solution.

Concentrations can be expressed as a fraction (mg/mL), a ratio (1:1000), or a percentage (60%). When a pharmacy technician receives an order to prepare a solution, the following terms are used to determine what is required to compound:

- **final strength (FS)**: the strength of the final solution
- **final volume (FV)**: the volume of the final solution
- **initial strength (IS)**: the strength of the original product used to prepare the final solution
- **initial volume (IV)**: the volume of the original product used to prepare the final solution
- **final weight (FW)**: for solids, the strength of the final solution
- **initial weight (IW)**: for solids, the strength of the original product used to prepare the final solution

The formula for compounding is:

*IV (or IW)× IS = FV (or FW) × FS*

Three formulas are used to calculate concentrations by percentages. Percentages are changed to equivalent decimal fractions by dropping the percent sign (%) and dividing the expressed numerator by a fraction. The formulas are:

- **Weight/weight (w/w%)** is the number of grams of a mass solute dissolved in 100 grams of a total mass solution, or vehicle base. The weight—not the volume—of each chemical is determined.

  w/w% = (weight of solute/weight of solution) × 100

- **Volume/volume (v/v%)** is the number of milliliters of volume solute dissolved in 100 milliliters of volume solution, or vehicle base. The volume of each chemical—not the weight—is determined.

  v/v% = (volume of solute in mg/volume of solution in mL) × 100

- **Weight/volume (w/v%)** is the number of grams of mass solute dissolved in 100 milliliters of a volume solution, or vehicle base. This formula is used when a solid is dissolved into a liquid.

  w/v% = (weight of solute/volume of solution) × 100

## QUICK REVIEW QUESTIONS

5.  What is the w/v% if 42 g of potassium is added to 1 L of sodium chloride?

    A)  0.42%

    B)  4.2%

    C)  42%

    D)  420%

6.  If 15 g of hydrocortisone is added to 120 g of cold cream, what is the w/w% of hydrocortisone?

    A)  0.125%

    B)  1.25%

    C)  12.5%

    D)  125%

## Ratio Strength

Many solutions require only a very tiny amount of a drug in order to be effective. When this happens, the **ratio strength** will be indicated on the product labeling; it is also known as **strength-to-weight ratio**. It is written using a slash (/) or colon (:). For example, ratio strength may be expressed in three concentrations: 1 mL/100 mL, 1 mL/1000 mL, and 1 mL/10,000 mL. Ratio strength may also be described as 1:100, 1:1000, and 1:10,000.

To calculate ratio strength in percentage, it's easiest to set up a proportion with the active ingredient on the top and the inactive ingredient on the bottom.

- In calculations, ratio strength is expressed as 1 in $x$, the corresponding fraction having a numerator of 1.

- In the ratio strength, the 1 in the ratio must correspond to the drug (active ingredient), not the solution.

- For w/v ratio strengths, volume is expressed in mL and weight in grams.

7. If 5 g of a product contains 250 mg of sodium chloride, what is the ratio strength?

   A) 1:25

   B) 1:20

   C) 1:10

   D) 1:5

## Stock Solutions

**Stock solutions** are solutions that have concentrations that are already known and are prepared for stock by the pharmacy staff for ease in dispensing. Rather than keeping large amounts of a solution in the pharmacy, concentrated amounts are kept. Then, the stock solutions can be **diluted** to the desired concentration needed for the preparation of the final product.

Stock solutions are prepared on a **weight-in-volume basis** so that other, weaker solutions can be made from them. Weight-in-volume is normally expressed as a percentage or ratio strength and is calculated with the following formula:

$$IV \ (or \ IW) \times IS = FV \ (or \ FW) \times FS.$$

 **HELPFUL HINT**

When solutions are diluted, the concentration of the drug decreases and the volume increases.

## QUICK REVIEW QUESTION

8. To what volume must 500 mL of a 10% w/v solution be diluted to produce a 2.5% solution?

   A) 1,000 mL

   B) 1,500 mL

   C) 2,000 mL

   D) 2,500 mL

## Liquid Dilutions

Liquid solutions are normally diluted with water or saline solutions. These solvents are called **diluents**. **Dilutions** represent the parts of the concentrate in total mass or volume.

The formula for dilution is $C_1 V_1 = C_2 V_2$ where:

- $C_1$ = concentration of stock solution
- $V_1$ = volume of stock solution needed to make the new solution
- $C_2$ = final concentration of new solution
- $V_2$ = final volume of new solution

Note: This formula can apply to weight instead of volume.

## QUICK REVIEW QUESTIONS

9. Mary has 40 L of a 5 g/L solution. To this solution, she adds 10 L. What is the final concentration of the solution?

    A) 1 g/L

    B) 3 g/L

    C) 4 g/L

    D) 2.5 g/L

10. Mark has 5 L of a 10 g/L solution. He needs to add 15 L to this solution to make the needed concentration. What is the final concentration of the solution? (Hint: we are looking for $C_2$.)

    A) 1.25 g/L

    B) 2.5 g/L

    C) 7.5 g/L

    D) 15 g/L

## Solid Dilutions

**Solids**, such as ointments, creams, and lotions, can also be diluted with another solid. This is normally done with the **trituration method**. In trituration, a potent drug powder is diluted with an inert diluent powder (usually lactose). The dilution occurs proportionally by weight. A weighable portion, or **aliquot**, of the mixture contains the desired amount of substance.

The formula used for dilution of solids by trituration is:

$$\text{weight of drug in} \frac{\text{trituration}}{\text{weight of trituration}} = \frac{\text{weight of drug in aliquot}}{\text{weight of aliquot}}$$

## QUICK REVIEW QUESTION

11. To determine the weight of the diluent needed to prepare the trituration after solving the formula, a pharmacy technician must

    A) subtract the weight of the drug being used for trituration by the trituration weight.

    B) multiply the weight of the drug being used for trituration by the trituration weight.

    C) divide the weight of the drug being used for trituration by the trituration weight.

    D) add the weight of the drug being used for trituration by the trituration weight.

## Alligations

Pharmacy alligation (also known as *"Tic-Tac-Toe"* math) is a shortcut for solving algebra problems. It is mainly used as an alternative to standard algebra when calculating the volumes for a compound made from different strengths of a similar chemical.

The easiest way to learn how to use alligation is to work through a sample problem.

A prescription order has arrived for 500 mL of a 12% solution. The pharmacy stocks the solution needed in 1 gallon of 30% solution and 1 gallon of 10% solution. You must mix the two solutions together to prepare a custom compound of the ordered volume. How much of the 30% solution will you need?

**Alligation Solution:**

Step 1: Draw a tic-tac-toe grid and put **higher % strength** in the top left square, **desired % strength** in the middle square, and **lower % strength** in the bottom left square:

|  |  |  |
|---|---|---|
| **30** |  |  |
|  | **12** |  |
| **10** |  |  |

Step 2: Calculate the difference between the bottom left number and the middle number going up diagonally, and also the difference from the top left and middle number going down diagonally (ignore any negatives). Then add up those two numbers to get 20. This sum becomes the "parts" needed to work with.

|  |  |  |  |
|---|---|---|---|
| **30** |  | <u>**2**</u> |  |
|  | **12** |  | **2 + 18 = 20 parts** |
| **10** |  | <u>**18**</u> |  |

Step 3: Now, divide the needed volume by the total parts: 500 mL ÷ 20 parts = 25 mL per part.

Step 4: On the grid, multiply the numbers in the right column by the milliliters per part to find the final volume.

|  |  |  |
|---|---|---|
| **30** |  | <u>**2 × 25 = 50 mL**</u> |
|  | **12** |  |
| **10** |  | <u>**18 × 25 = 450 mL**</u> |

50 mL of the 30% solution is needed.

## Alligation:

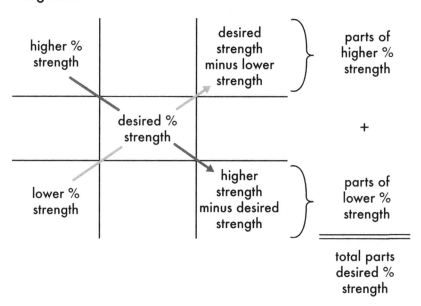

*Figure 4.1. Alligations*

### Algebraic Solution:

Let *x* = the amount of the 30% solution. Then 500 − *x* = the amount of the 10% solution, because they both must add up to 500 mL.

Now, fill out this chart:

| | Amount | % | Total | |
|---|---|---|---|---|
| **30% strength** | *x* | 0.30 | 0.3*x* | **multiply across** |
| **10% strength** | 500 − *x* | 0.10 | 0.10(500 − *x*) | **multiply across** |
| **Total (What we want)** | 500 | 0.12 | 60 | **multiply across** |
| | **Add down** | | **Add down: 0.3x + 0.10(500 − x) = 60; solve.** | |

Now solve for *x*, which is the amount of the 30% solution.

0.3*x* + 0.10(500 − *x*) = 60

0.3*x* + 50 − 0.10*x* = 60

0.2*x* = 10

**x = 50 mL**

## QUICK REVIEW QUESTION

**12.** A prescription for a 30 g tube of 2% hydrocortisone needs to be made from a 1% solution and a 2.5% solution. Using alligation, how much of each available product is needed to prepare this prescription?

    **A)** 1 g of 1% and 2.5 g of 2%

    **B)** 10 g of 1% and 20 g of 2.5%

    **C)** 15 g of 1% and 15 g of 2.5%

    **D)** 20 g of 1% and 10 g of 2.5%

## Pediatric Dosages

**Pediatric** refers to any patient eighteen years old or younger. Because infants and children cannot tolerate adult doses of drugs, drugs given to pediatric patients are dosed based on the child's age and weight. There are several methods for calculating pediatric dosages. The most accurate way is by weight: kilogram or pound. Pediatric dosages can also be calculated by body surface area (BSA) and age. Charts called **nomograms** are used to determine BSA by square meters according to height and weight.

 **HELPFUL HINT**

The most commonly used rule is Clark's rule. For Clark's rule, always use the weight of the child in pounds, not kilograms.

It is important to emphasize that not all drugs can be given to children, even with changes in dosage strength. Because of severe side effects or because the drug has not been tested on children, certain drugs are not to be given to children at all. It is also important to stress how crucial it is to be accurate in calculating dosage strengths for children. Most medication errors occur due to mistakes made in pediatric dosing. A single mistake in the placement of a decimal point can cause injury or death in children.

*The Pediatric Dosage Handbook* is one reference tool used in the pharmacy setting for resources on pediatric dosing; it includes **manufacturer packaging**, labeling information, and requirements. It is also important to state that if the technician has any questions, he or she should ask the pharmacist-in-charge or a supervisor for verification of correct dosing.

Three formulas are used for calculating dosage for infants and children. The formulas are Clark's rule, Young's rule, and Fried's rule. Fried's Rule is the least common calculation as it is only used for pediatric patients under twenty-four months of age.

- Clark's rule: child's dose = $\dfrac{\text{weight of the child}}{150} \times$ average adult dose

- Young's rule: child's dose = adult dose $\times \dfrac{\text{age}}{\text{age} + 12}$

- Fried's rule: child's dose = $\dfrac{\text{child's age in months}}{150} \times$ adult dose

Another way to calculate dosage strengths is by using a nomogram. A nomogram is a graphic representation of several lines that *connect* two known values on two lines and an unknown value at the point of intersection with another line. In pharmacy, nomograms show height, weight, and BSA in graph form with a graphic value of dosage values based on children of the same height and weight. Doses are then calculated based on normal adult doses by multiplying the BSA in square meters by the dose ordered.

The formula for calculation using a nonogram is: weight per dose × BSA = desired dose

## Example for a child who is 52 inches tall and weighs 90 pounds

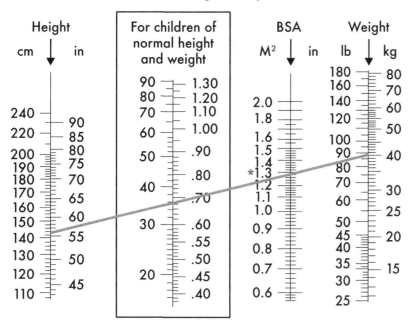

*Figure 4.2. Pediatric Nomogram*

## Body Surface Area Nomogram

### Body Surface Area from Height and Weight

$$BSA = W^{0.425} \times H^{0.725} \times 71.84$$

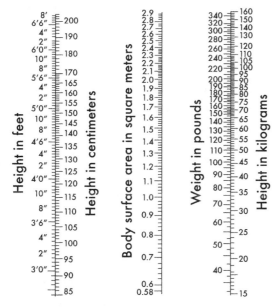

In the above formula, weight is in kgm and height is in cm, giving body surface area in cm².

*Figure 4.3. Body Surface Area Nomogram*

13. If a physician orders Cefzil for a 38 lb child, what would be the pediatric dose given if the adult dose of Cefzil is 600 mg q 24 h? (Use Clark's rule.)

    **A)** 85.4 mg

    **B)** 150.2 mg

    **C)** 152 mg

    **D)** 250 mg

14. A physician orders Zyrtec 0.1 mg/kg daily for a child who weighs 70 lbs. What is the correct pediatric dose for the patient?

    **A)** 5.5 mg daily

    **B)** 3.18 mg daily

    **C)** 2.75 mg daily

    **D)** 1.25 mg daily

# Compounding

**Compounding** is the personalized preparation, from one or more ingredients, of a prescribed medication that is not commercially available. There are a wide range of medications that can be compounded. Some can be as simple as adding product flavoring to a child's antibiotic to improve taste, while other product formulations need to be precisely calculated into patient-specific customized dosage forms.

## Non-Sterile Compounding

**Non-sterile compounding** (also called **extemporaneous compounding**) refers to the compounding of two or more ingredients that a patient can swallow, drink, insert, or apply topically. Some circumstances that would require compounding follow.

- Commercially unavailable products: Topical hormonal therapies, veterinary preparations, specialty dermatologic products that are applied topically, and patient-specific rectal or vaginal compounds all may require compounding.

- Specialized dosage strengths: If a patient-specific dosage or strength of a preparation is needed that is not commercially available, the pharmacy technician may need to compound it.

- Product flavoring: If the taste of a medication affects compliance, compounding may be necessary.

- A different dosage form is needed: If a patient cannot take capsules or tablets, then a liquid formulation may be compounded.

According to USP 795, any equipment or supplies used to compound MUST:

- reduce ingredients to the smallest particle size.

**HELPFUL HINT**

The FDA requires that non-sterile compounding must adhere to the standards of USP Chapter 795 and follow DEA guidelines. The DEA requires specific compounding record logs for narcotics, a recording of inventory after each batch, and a record kept by the pharmacist regarding any waste.

- ensure the solution has no visible undissolved matter when dispensed.
- make sure preparations are similarly structured to ensure uniform final distribution.

Some preparations are made to the patient's order, while other formulations may be commonly prescribed by a physician. If the latter is the case, the pharmacy has a **master formula record**, or recipes of frequently used compounding formulas and recordkeeping. Some formulations that are frequently prescribed may be made in bulk so the product can be dispensed to the patient in a timely manner.

Any time a compounded medication is prepared, it must be verified by a pharmacist. It also must be recorded in a **compounding log** with the name of products used, lot numbers, expiration and beyond-use dates, quantity made, and amount of ingredients used (lot numbers and expiration dates on packaging are always grouped together). The initials of the technician who prepared the medication and the pharmacist who verified it are required as well. It is then filed as a permanent record.

## QUICK REVIEW QUESTION

**15.** Which of the following situations would NOT require non-sterile compounding?

**A)** A patient is allergic to an inactive ingredient in a commercially made topical cream.

**B)** A patient has a prescription for an enteric-coated tablet that is small and easy to swallow.

**C)** A child refuses to take an antibiotic because of its bad taste.

**D)** A physician prescribes a drug in which a dosage form is not currently manufactured.

## Tools for Compounding

For measuring and weighing, technicians use different tools. **Class A balances** are required in all pharmacies and must be inspected and meet the requirements of the National Bureau of Standards (NBS). A Class A balance is a two-pan torsion type with internal and external weights. It has a capacity of 120 mg and a sensitivity of 6 mg. **Counter balances** are less accurate than Class A balances. They have a limit of 5 kg and a sensitivity of 100 mg.

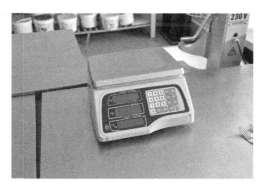

*Figure 4.4. Counter Balance*

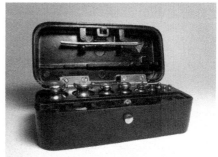

*Figure 4.5. Class A Balance*

In addition, **weighing boats** and **glassine paper** are flexible containers used for holding liquids and solids that are weighed on the balances.

**Weights** are usually made of brass or polished metal and must be maintained and handled properly. Sets generally contain cylindrical weights ranging from 1 – 50 g and fractional weights of 10 – 500 mg. The weights should be calibrated annually to ensure accuracy. **Forceps** should be used when picking up weights to prevent damage.

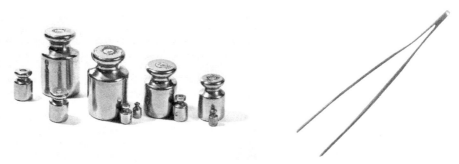

Figure 4.6. Weights

Figure 4.7. Forceps

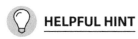

**HELPFUL HINT**

Measurement should be taken at the bottom of the meniscus.

**Conical graduated cylinders** are used for measuring liquids and pouring due to their circular design. **Cylindrical graduated cylinders** are also used for measuring liquids but have a narrow design. The **meniscus** is the curved upper surface of a liquid in a container: it is curved in if the liquid wets the walls and curved out if it does not.

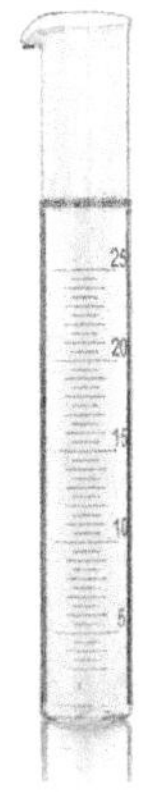

Some other common tools and equipment used for extemporaneous compounding include the following:

- **suppository molds**: Plastic or metal, these molds are used to form the suppository after it has been prepared.

- **capsule-filling equipment**: This mechanical device fills the gelatin capsules with powder.

Figure 4.8. Cylindrical Graduated Cylinder

- **tablet mold**: Tablet molds are small, usually cylindrical, molded, or compressed disks of different sizes. They contain a diluent—usually made of dextrose or a mixture of lactose and powdered sucrose—and a moistening agent or diluted alcohol.

- **compounding or ointment slab**: This slab is a plate made of glass or porcelain and used for geometric dilution and mixing. It can be easily cleaned.

- **compounding spatula**: This tool is made of flexible rubber or metal and is used to mix and shear ointments and creams.

- **blenders and mixers**: These common devices can be used for mixing as well.

- A **mortar and pestle** is a tool that has been used for centuries in pharmacy. It is used to grind and crush, or **levigate**, ingredients into a fine paste. These tools are usually made of wood, ceramics, or stone.

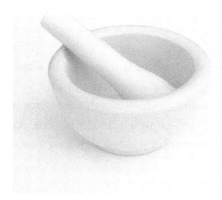

*Figure 4.9. Mortar and Pestle (ceramic)*

## QUICK REVIEW QUESTION

**16.** Which compound can be made using a mold?

**A)** a capsule

**B)** a tablet

**C)** a solution

**D)** a lotion

## Compounding Procedures

Common preparations that can be made by extemporaneous compounding include the following:

- **ointment**: an oily preparation that is normally medicated and applied topically

- **cream**: a thick or semisolid preparation applied topically

- **paste**: a thick, soft, and moist substance usually produced by mixing dry ingredients with a liquid

- **oil-in-water emulsion**: a diffusion (droplets) of one liquid in another, impassible liquid

- **solution**: a liquid preparation of one or more soluble chemical substances that are usually dissolved in water

- **suspension**: a preparation of finely divided, undissolved drugs or powders distributed in a liquid medium

- **capsule**: a solid encapsulated in gelatin

- **tablet**: a compressed solid dosage unit

- **troche** (lozenge): a molded solid meant to dissolve in the mouth
- **suppository**: a solid preparation in either conical or cylindrical shape that is inserted into the rectum or vagina to dissolve

Compounding requires precision and attention to detail. Mistakes can result in medications that are ineffective or even harmful to the patient. Each pharmacy will have its own policies and procedures for compounding, so only general guidelines are discussed here.

Solutions and suspensions are some of the most commonly compounded medications. In a solution, a **solute** is dissolved in a **solvent**. Solutions should always be mixed thoroughly to ensure that all of the solute has been dissolved. **Precipitation**—solids falling out of a solution—are usually a sign that the solution has not been mixed completely or has been compounded incorrectly. Unexpected discoloration can be another sign that a medication has been compounded incorrectly.

**Reconstitution** is the process of adding a precise amount of sterile water to the powdered form of a drug to form a suspension. Reconstituted suspensions must be shaken thoroughly by the patient before use to ensure that the drug has been distributed evenly throughout the water.

Tablets are made by mixing the active drug with a **base** (usually a sugar, like dextrose) and other additives. The mixture is pressed into tablets using a mold. Capsules are made similarly by measuring the appropriate amount of a powdered mixture and using a capsule-filling machine. For both tablets and capsules, USP 795 states that they cannot weigh less than 90 percent or more than 110 percent of the calculated unit weight.

## QUICK REVIEW QUESTION

17. A formulation where an undissolved drug or powder is distributed in a liquid medium is what?

   **A)** a cream

   **B)** a suppository

   **C)** a suspension

   **D)** an ointment

## Sig Codes and Abbreviations

Pharmacy abbreviations—also called **sig codes**—are used when preparing medical prescriptions and hospital medication orders. These codes are extremely important to the pharmacy technician and must be known in order for the technician to decipher important instructions, measurements, and times needed for a patient's medications.

## TABLE 4.4. Common Sig Codes

| Abbreviation | Meaning | Category |
|---|---|---|
| $\dot{\bar{\imath}}$ | one | measurement |
| $\bar{s}$ | without | other |
| $\ddot{\bar{s}}s$; ss | one-half | measurement |
| a.a., aa | of each | measurement |
| a.c. | before meals | time |
| ad | to, up to | measurement |
| a.d. | right ear | route of administration |
| ad lib | at one's pleasure | time |
| agit. | shake, stir | other |
| alt. h. | every other hour | time |
| a.m. | morning | time |
| amp. | ampule | other |
| app. | apply | route of administration |
| aq, aqua | water | drug form |
| aq. ad | add water up to | measurement |
| a.s., a.l. | left ear | route of administration |
| A.T.C. | around the clock | time |
| a.u. | both ears | route of administration |
| b.i.d., b.d. | twice daily | time |
| b.m. | bowel movement | other |
| bol. | bolus | other |
| B.S. | blood sugar | other |
| B.S.A. | body surface area | measurement |
| c | with | other |
| cap or caps | capsules | drug form |
| cc | cubic centimeter | measurement |
| comp. | compound | drug form |
| cr., crm. | cream | drug form |
| D5NS | dextrose 5% in sodium chloride solution | drug |

*continued on next page*

## TABLE 4.4. Common Sig Codes *(continued)*

| Abbreviation | Meaning | Category |
|---|---|---|
| D5W | dextrose 5% in water | drug |
| D.A.W. | dispense as written | other |
| dc, D/C, disc. | discontinue | other |
| dil. | dilute | measurement |
| disp. | dispense | other |
| div. | divide | measurement |
| d.t.d. | dispense such doses | other |
| D.W. | distilled water | drug form |
| elix. | elixir | drug form |
| emuls. | emulsion | drug form |
| e.t. | expired time | time |
| ex aq. | in water | other |
| fl., fld. | fluid | drug form |
| fl. oz. | fluid ounce | measurement |
| g, G, gm | gram | measurement |
| gtt(s) | drop(s) | measurement |
| h, hr. | hour | time |
| h.s. | at bedtime | time |
| i.d. | intradermal | other |
| i.m., IM | intramuscularly | route of administration |
| inj. | inject | route of administration |
| i.v., IV | intravenously | route of administration |
| IVP | IV push | route of administration |
| IVPB | IV piggyback | route of administration |
| l., L. | liter | measurement |
| LCD | coal tar solution | drug form |
| lin. | liniment | drug form |
| liq. | liquid | drug form |
| lot. | lotion | drug form |
| mcg | microgram | measurement |
| mEq | milliequivalent | measurement |

| Abbreviation | Meaning | Category |
| --- | --- | --- |
| mg | milligram | measurement |
| min. | minute | time |
| mist. | mixture | drug form |
| mL | milliliter | measurement |
| neb., nebul. | nebulizer | other |
| NMT | not more than | other |
| noct. | at night | time |
| non rep. | do not repeat | time |
| NR | no refill | other |
| NS | normal saline, sodium chloride | drug form |
| ½NS | half strength normal saline | drug form |
| NTE | not to exceed | other |
| o.d. | right eye | route of administration |
| o.s., o.l. | left eye | route of administration |
| o.u. | both eyes | route of administration |
| oz | ounce | measurement |
| p.c. | after food, after meals | time |
| per | by | other |
| p.m. | afternoon, evening | time |
| p.o. | by mouth | route of administration |
| p.r. | rectally | route of administration |
| prn | as needed | route of administration |
| pulv. | pulverized | other |
| q | each, every | time |
| q.a.m. | every morning | time |
| q.d. | every day | time |
| q.h. | every hour | time |
| q.h.s. | every night at bedtime | time |
| q.i.d. | four times daily | time |
| q.o.d. | every other day | time |
| q.s. | a sufficient quantity | measurement |
| R | rub | other |

*continued on next page*

## TABLE 4.4. Common Sig Codes *(continued)*

| Abbreviation | Meaning | Category |
|---|---|---|
| rep., rept. | repeat | other |
| RL, R/L | Ringer's lactated | drug form |
| SC, subc, subQ, subcut | subcutaneous | route of administration |
| sig | write on label | other |
| SL | sublingual | route of administration |
| sol. | solution | drug form |
| SR, XL, XR | slow release/extended release | drug form |
| ss | one-half | other |
| stat. | immediately | time |
| sup. | suppository | drug form |
| susp. | suspension | drug form |
| syr. | syrup | drug form |
| tab. | tablet | drug form |
| talc. | talcum | drug form |
| tbsp | tablespoonful | measurement |
| t.i.d., tid | three times daily | time |
| t.i.w. | three times a week | time |
| top. | topically | route of administration |
| TPN | total parenteral nutrition | other |
| troche | lozenge | drug form |
| tsp | teaspoonful | measurement |
| u.d., utd., ut. dict. | as directed | other |
| ung., oint. | ointment | drug form |
| USP | United States Pharmacopeia | other |
| vag. | vaginally | route of administration |
| w | with | other |
| w/o, wo | without | other |
| X | times | other |
| y.o., Y.O. | years old | other |

## QUICK REVIEW QUESTIONS

**18.** What does "Take 1 tab. q.i.d. prn pain" mean?

   **A)** Take 1 teaspoonful every 4 hours as needed for pain.

   **B)** Take 1 tablet every day as needed for pain.

   **C)** Take 1 tablet four times daily as needed for pain.

   **D)** Take 1 tablespoonful every day as needed for pain.

**19.** What is the translation of "Instill 1 gtt in o.u. b.d."?

   **A)** Instill 1 drop in the left ear twice daily.

   **B)** Instill 1 drop in both eyes twice daily.

   **C)** Instill 1 drop in the left eye twice daily.

   **D)** Instill 1 drop in both ears twice daily.

## Drug Administration Equipment

After the completion of drug preparation, it is critical to make sure the patient understands how to administer or self-administer the medication correctly. For some medications, this may require the technician to provide **administration equipment** appropriate to the specific patient and medication form. Some common examples of this equipment are below.

- **Oral syringes** are used to measure and dispense oral liquids to children or adults who cannot swallow solid drug forms. They are also used for liquid measurements in small doses (under a teaspoon).

- **Droppers** are used to administer smaller volumes of liquid to infants and children.

- **Medication cups** are used to measure larger liquid dosages.

- **Pill splitters** are devices used to cut solid forms, like tablets, into pieces.

- **Spacers** are tubes attached to inhalers that ensure the patient receives an accurate dose of a medication. They are usually given to children, the elderly, or anyone who cannot use an inhaler properly.

- **Unit dose drug packages** are prepackaged with a single dose of a drug.

- **Syringes and needles** are used to measure and dispense drug medications given parenterally, including IM, IV, ID, and sub-Q. Types of syringes include standard (for volumes over 1 mL), tuberculin syringes (for volumes less than 1 mL), and insulin syringes (which have measurements marked in units).

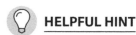

**HELPFUL HINT**

**Scored** tablets are marked with lines that equally divide the tablet into two or four parts.

**HELPFUL HINT**

Spacers may be covered under some insurance plans, but a provider will need to prescribe it.

→
CONTINUE

**20.** A pharmacy technician is dispensing an antibiotic oral suspension for an infant. If the dosage is 10 mL, what administration equipment should the technician include?

**A)** oral syringe

**B)** medication cup

**C)** syringe

**D)** unit dose packaging

# National Drug Code Numbers and Lot Numbers

In 1972, the **Drug Listing Act** implemented the use of **national drug codes (NDCs)**. Every drug has a ten or eleven-digit NDC divided into three sections. The first section, which consists of four or five numbers, is the labeler or manufacturer's code and is provided by the FDA. The second is the product code and it specifies the product or drug. The third is the package code and represents the size and type of the product. If the NDC has two asterisks (*) at the end of the package number, it means that the product is a bulk, raw, or non-formulated controlled substance.

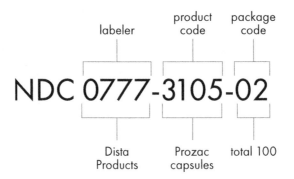

Figure 4.10. NDC Number

Federal regulations state that all manufactured drugs must have **lot numbers**, which are assigned by the manufacturer. Batches of drugs that are manufactured together have the same lot numbers. This allows manufacturers to easily recall specific batches of drugs. Lot numbers are comprised of all numbers, or all letters, or a combination of numbers and letters.

**HELPFUL HINT**

When a drug has been recalled, the pharmacy will be given a lot number to be pulled from shelves.

**QUICK REVIEW QUESTION**

**21.** What does the third section of an NDC number represent?

**A)** package size

**B)** the manufacturer

**C)** the dosage form

**D)** the strength of the medication

## Disposing of Medications

To effectively manage the drug inventory inside of a pharmacy, a technician will check for expired drugs, prescriptions not picked up by patients, or drugs that have not been prescribed. These drugs must be properly disposed of.

The technician must maintain the inventory of stocked drugs on the shelf by consistently checking for **expired medications** to ensure the patient is receiving a quality product. Three months before the drug is due to expire, the pharmacy technician marks the stock bottle, based on the pharmacy's procedure, to alert the staff the drug will be expiring soon. (Many pharmacies use a brightly colored sticker with the date of expiration.)

When checking expiration dates, if the date on the stock bottle states 5/20, the medication will expire on the last day of May in the year 2020. If the expiration date states 5/15/20, the medication will expire on May 15, 2020. Expired medications must be completely removed from the shelf a month before the expiration date.

Although pharmacies may have different inspection policies and procedures, pharmacy technicians must check the inventory for expired medications monthly. While they are checking for expired drugs to pull, technicians also ensure that the stock is rotated correctly. This task includes making sure the stock bottle with the earliest expiration date is placed in front of the other stock bottles on the shelf and that open bottles are marked so the staff does not open a new bottle before the open bottle is finished.

Once expired drugs are pulled from the shelves, they are then stored separately from other active drugs in the pharmacy to prevent the pharmacy staff from accidently dispensing them. The drugs are then disposed of based on the policy of the pharmacy.

If patients do not pick up their medication within seven days of the original fill, the pharmacy should attempt to contact them and remind them about the filled medication. When all communication efforts have been exhausted, the pharmacy can note that the order has been categorized as a **patient decline**. The technician can then return the drug item to stock. Special-order items can be returned to the manufacturer for credit and the medication claim is canceled for third-party billing purposes.

**Excess stock** should be returned to the manufacturer, often for full or partial credit. Controlled substances have restricted disposal procedures which require a pharmacist. (See chapter 2 for information on the disposal of controlled substances.)

## QUICK REVIEW QUESTION

22. Stock bottles of expiring medications are removed from the shelf

   A) one month before expiring.

   B) two months before expiring.

   C) three months before expiring.

   D) two weeks before expiring.

1. **C)**

   $3 \text{ tbsp} \times \dfrac{15 \text{ mL}}{1 \text{ tbsp}} = \textbf{45 mL}$

2. **C)**

   $4 \text{ oz} \times \dfrac{30 \text{ g}}{1 \text{ oz}} = \textbf{120 g}$

3. **C)**

   part = whole × percent = 48 × 0.75 = **36**

4. **B)**

   Identify the formula and variables.

   specific gravity = $\dfrac{\text{weight (g)}}{\text{volume (mL)}}$

   weight =45 g

   volume = 500 mL

   Solve for specific gravity.

   specific gravity = $\dfrac{45 \text{ g}}{500 \text{ mL}}$ = **0.09 g/mL**

5. **B)**

   Identify the variables and formula (weight must be in **grams** and volume in **mL**). Note that the solute is the potassium, and the vehicle base is the sodium chloride.

   weight of solute = 42 g

   volume of vehicle base (in mL)=1 L=1000 mL

   $\dfrac{w}{v}\% = \dfrac{\text{weight of solute (g)}}{\text{volume of vehical base (mL)}} \times 100$

   Solve for w/v %.

   $\dfrac{w}{v}\% = \dfrac{42 \text{ g}}{1{,}000 \text{ mL}}$ = 0.042 × 100 = **4.2%**

6. **C)**

   Identify variables and formula. Note that the solute is the hydrocortisone, and the vehicle base is the cold cream.

   volume of solute = 15 g

   volume of vehicle base =120 g

   w/w% = $\dfrac{\text{volume of solute}}{\text{volume of vehicle base}} \times 100$

   Solve for w/w %.

   $\dfrac{w}{w}\% = \dfrac{15 \text{ g}}{120 \text{ g}}$ = 0.125 × 100 = **12.5%**

7. **B)**

   Convert the 250 mg of sodium chloride (the active ingredient) into grams, so the units will match.

   250 mg = 0.25 g

   Set up a proportion with the drug on the top and the sodium chloride solution on the bottom.

   $\dfrac{0.25 \text{ g}}{5 \text{ g}} = \dfrac{1}{x}$

   Cross-multiply and solve for the ratio strength, which will be a number greater than 1. Then describe ratio strength in a ratio with 1 corresponding to the active ingredient amount.

$0.25x = 5$

$x = 20$

**1:20**

8. **B)**

Identify variables.

$x$ = volume of sterile water to be added) $C_1$ = concentration of stock solution (actual drug) = 10%

$V_1$ = volume of stock solution needed to make new solution = 500 L

$C_2$ = final concentration of new solution = 2.5%

$V_2$ = final volume of new solution = (500 + $x$) L

Plug the values in the appropriate formula. Isolate $x$ to get solution.

$C_1V_1 = C_2V_2$

$0.10 \times 500 = 0.025(500 + x)$

$50 = 12.5 + 0.025x$

$0.025x = 50 - 12.5 = 37.5$

$x = \frac{37.5}{0.025}$

**$x = 1500$ mL**

9. **C)**

Identify variables.

$x$ = final concentration of new solution

$C_1$ = concentration of stock solution (actual drug) = 5 g/L

$V_1$ = volume of stock solution needed to make new solution = 40 L

$C_2$ = final concentration of new solution = $x$ g/L

$V_2$ = final volume of new solution = 40 L + 10 L = 50 L

Plug the values in the appropriate formula. Isolate $x$ to get the solution.

$C_1V_1 = C_2V_2$

$5(40) = x(50)$

$200 = x(50)$

$200 = 50x$

**$x = 4$ g/L**

10. **B)**

Identify variables.

$x$ = final concentration of new solution in g/L

$C_1$ = concentration of stock solution (actual drug) = 10 g/L

$V_1$ = volume of stock solution needed to make new solution = 5 L

$C_2$ = final concentration of new solution = $x$

$V_2$ = final volume of new solution = 5 L + 15 L = 20 L

Plug the values in the appropriate formula. Isolate $x$ to get the solution.

$C_1V_1 = C_2V_2$

$10(5) = 20(x)$

$50 = 20x$

$$x = \frac{50}{20}$$
$$x = 2.5 \text{ g/L}$$

11.   **A)**

Subtracting the weight of the drug being used for trituration by the trituration weight will determine the weight of the diluent.

12.   **B)**

**Alligation Solution:**

Step 1: Draw a tic-tac-toe grid and put **higher % strength** in the top left square, **desired % strength** in the middle square, and **lower % strength** in the bottom left square:

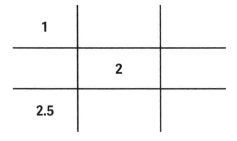

Step 2: Calculate the difference between the bottom left number and the middle number going up diagonally, and the difference from the top left and middle numbers going down diagonally (ignore any negatives). Then add up those two numbers to get 1.5. This sum becomes the "parts."

| 1 | | **0.5** |
|---|---|---|
| | 2 | |
| 2.5 | | **1** |

**0.5 + 1 = 1.5 parts**

Step 3: Now, divide the needed volume into the total parts: 30 g ÷ 1.5 parts = 20 g per part.

Step 4: On the grid, go back up to the parts and write the volume for each part.

| 1 | | **0.5 × 20 = 10 g** |
|---|---|---|
| | 2 | |
| 2.5 | | **1 × 20 = 20 g** |

So, 0.5 parts of the 1% solution × 20 g = **10 g**, and 1 part of the 2.5% solution × 20 g = **20 g.**

**Algebraic Solution:**

Let $x$ = the amount of the 1% solution. Then $30 - x$ = the amount of the 2.5% solution because they both have to add up to 30 g.

Now fill out this chart:

|  | Amount | % | Total |  |
|---|---|---|---|---|
| 1% strength | x | 0.01 | 0.01x | multiply across |
| 2.5% strength | 30 – x | 0.025 | 0.025(30 – x) | multiply across |
| Total (desired quantity) | 30 | 0.02 | .6 | multiply across |
|  | Add down |  | Add down: 0.01x + 0.025(30 – x) = 0.6; solve. |  |

Solve for x, which is the amount of the 1% solution.

$0.01x + 0.75 – 0.025X = 0.6$

$-0.015x = -0.15$

$x = 10$ g

Then, to get the 2.5% solution, subtract this from 30.

$30 – x =$ **20 g**

13. **C)**

Identify the formula and variables. (Note that the child's weight is already in pounds.)

$$\text{child's dose} = \frac{\text{weight of the child}}{150} \times \text{adult dose}$$

weight of the child = 38 lb

adult dose = 600 mg

Solve for child's dose.

$$\text{child's dose} = \frac{38}{150} \times 600 \text{ mg} = \textbf{152 mg}$$

14. **B)**

Multiply by conversion ratios to cancel out units until arriving at the needed units. (Recall that 1 kg ≈ 2.2 lb.)

$$\frac{0.1 \text{ mg}}{\text{kg}} \times \frac{1 \text{ kg}}{2.2 \text{ lb}} \times 70 \text{ lb} = \textbf{3.18 mg}$$

15. **B)**

A coated tablet would not be made using non-sterile compounding techniques.

16. **B)**

A tablet can be made using a mold.

17. **C)**

A suspension is a preparation of undissolved drugs or powders distributed in a liquid medium.

18. **C)**

   tab. = tablet

   q.i.d. = four times a day

   prn = as needed)

19. **B)**

   gtt (gutta) = drop

   o.u. (oculus uterque) = both eyes

   b.d. or b.i.d. (bis in die) = twice daily

20. **A)**

   An oral syringe should be used to measure and administer small amounts of an oral suspension to infants.

21. **A)**

   The third part of an NDC describes the package size.

22. **A)**

   Expiring medications should be removed from the shelf one month before the expiration date.

# 5 PTCB Practice Test

1. Salmeterol is used primarily to:
   A) prevent asthma attacks and bronchospasms.
   B) lower fevers and treat inflammation.
   C) treat autoimmune disorders.
   D) modulate estrogen levels.

2. The pharmacy receives the following prescription:

   > Spiriva Respimat, 1.25 mcg
   > Disp: one inhaler
   > Sig: 2 puffs BID

   How many days should the supply last if there are 60 metered doses in each inhaler?
   A) 15
   B) 30
   C) 45
   D) 60

3. If a drug's expiration date is written as June 2021, the last day the drug may be used is:
   A) May 31, 2021.
   B) June 1, 2021.
   C) June 30, 2021.
   D) July 1, 2021.

4. Which of the following generic medications can be substituted for Vasotec?
   A) atenolol
   B) metoprolol
   C) metronidazole
   D) enalapril

5. DEA Form 106 is used for:
   A) ordering and returning Schedule II drugs.
   B) theft or loss.
   C) DEA registration.
   D) destroying controlled substances.

6. A laminar flow hood in the pharmacy is designed to:
   A) provide filtered air directly over the work surface.
   B) be sterile on the inside.
   C) move air away from the work area.
   D) remove hazardous fumes from the work area.

7. All of the following information must be included on a Schedule II prescription hard copy EXCEPT:
   A) the manual signature of the physician.
   B) the patient's name and address.
   C) the prescriber's DEA number.
   D) the drug's NDC number.

8. A 2% dextrose stock solution and a 10% dextrose stock solution are being used to make 250 mL of a 5% dextrose solution. How many milliliters of the 10% solution should be used?

A) 50 mL

B) 31.25 mL

C) 93.75 mL

D) 145.8 mL

9. The generic name for Protonix is:

A) omeprazole.

B) esomeprazole.

C) pantoprazole.

D) lansoprazole.

10. Which auxiliary label should be affixed to a prescription bottle of metformin ER?

A) Do not chew or crush. Swallow whole.

B) Do not ingest any form of grapefruit.

C) Take medication on an empty stomach.

D) May cause drowsiness.

11. If 5 capsules of amoxicillin contain 2,500 mg of amoxicillin, how many capsules are required to fill a prescription for 50,000 mg?

A) 25

B) 50

C) 75

D) 100

12. Which of the following medications should be taken with food?

A) meloxicam

B) Fioricet

C) ondansetron

D) varenicline

13. The purpose of Tall Man lettering is to:

A) differentiate among LASA drugs.

B) ensure correct pronunciation of drug names.

C) prevent spelling errors.

D) speed up the prescription labeling process.

14. Which of the following medications is contraindicated for pregnant patients?

A) Humalog

B) chlorhexidine gluconate

C) tizanidine

D) warfarin

15. Which of the following is NOT a Schedule drug?

A) pregabalin

B) lorazepam

C) metronidazole

D) methylphenidate

16. Dr. Johnson became a physician in 1981. Which of the following could be her DEA number?

A) AJ1673929

B) BJ1673929

C) JB1673929

D) JA1673929

17. Which of the following is NOT a side effect of ciprofloxacin?

A) vomiting

B) diarrhea

C) constipation

D) headache

18. How long from the date it is written is a prescription for a noncontrolled substance valid?

A) 2 years

B) 1 year

C) 6 months

D) 30 days

19. Which health care professional does NOT have prescribing authority?

A) nurse practitioners

B) registered nurses

C) physicians

D) psychiatrists

20. A patient is taking hydrotussin, 2 teaspoons q 4 hrs as needed for cough. The doctor gave the patient 8 ounces of the hydrotussin. If the patient took the medication exactly as written, every 4 hours, how long would the 8-ounce bottle last?

A) 7 days

B) 6 days

C) 5 days

D) 4 days

21. A pharmacy technician should alert the pharmacist to counsel a patient who has presented a prescription for:

A) doxycycline for a 4-year-old.

B) omeprazole for a 70-year-old.

C) famotidine for a 16-year-old.

D) 81 mg aspirin for a 30-year-old.

22. Which of the following is used for weighing non-sterile compound ingredients?

A) counter balance

B) compounding slab

C) suppository mold

D) mortar and pestle

23. Which of the following medications does NOT have edema as a potential side effect?

A) sertraline

B) lisinopril

C) amlodipine

D) sildenafil

24. Which of the following is a common side effect of ACE inhibitors?

A) cough

B) weight gain

C) weight loss

D) drowsiness

25. A pharmacy receives the following prescription:

Norco 5/325
Sig: 1 tab PO q 4 – 6 hours PRN × 10 days

How many tablets will be needed to fill this prescription?

A) 40

B) 60

C) 120

D) 240

26. A prescription is written for amoxicillin 250-mg capsules × 2 BID × 10 days. If the pharmacy only has 500-mg amoxicillin capsules in stock, how many capsules should be dispensed?

A) 10

B) 20

C) 40

D) 80

27. Which of the following drugs does NOT have a warning for patients under 18 years old?

A) paroxetine

B) aspirin

C) amoxicillin

D) escitalopram

28. The pharmacy receives the following prescription:

Lortab 7.5 mg
Dispense: #12
Sig: T PO q 4 – 6 hours PRN

Which of the following drug forms will the pharmacy technician dispense?

A) capsule

B) syrup

C) tablet

D) lozenge

29. Orphan drugs are developed for:

A) children with autoimmune conditions.

B) management of chronic respiratory conditions.

C) treatment of rare diseases.

D) replacement of high-cost brand-name drugs.

30. A patient taking which of the following medications should be counseled to avoid taking the medication with grapefruit?

A) lovastatin

B) citalopram

C) esomeprazole

D) furosemide

31. The abbreviation *rep, rept means:*
    A) no refill.
    B) label.
    C) as needed.
    D) repeat.

32. A prescription is written for pravastatin 60 mg tab qhs × 30 days. Pravastatin is only dispensed in 20 mg, 40 mg, and 80 mg, and each tablet is scored so it can be split in half. How many tablets are needed to fill this prescription?
    A) 30
    B) 45
    C) 60
    D) 63

33. Ondansetron is prescribed for:
    A) pain.
    B) diabetes.
    C) stomach acid.
    D) nausea.

34. A prescription contains the code DAW-1. The pharmacy technician should:
    A) dispense a generic substitute.
    B) dispense the name-brand medication written on the prescription.
    C) call the prescriber to confirm which generic should be substituted.
    D) call the patient's insurance company before dispensing the medication.

35. NDC numbers include all of the following information EXCEPT the:
    A) manufacturer's name.
    B) drug's name.
    C) package size.
    D) drug's expiration date.

36. Which of the following symptoms is NOT a common potential side effect of prednisone?
    A) headache
    B) dizziness
    C) blurred vision
    D) weight loss

37. Which of the following could be the DEA number for a manufacturer of Schedule II controlled substances?
    A) E97548398
    B) X99384758
    C) A91627833
    D) R96059489

38. Which of the following is on a patient's compounding label?
    A) physician's DEA number
    B) patient's Social Security number
    C) patient's allergies
    D) quantity

39. A pharmacy technician is compounding a prescription and mistakenly over-dilutes the compound. What should the technician do next?
    A) properly dispose of the compound and start the compounding process from the beginning
    B) figure out how much of the solute is needed to prepare the proper concentration and add it to the compound
    C) adjust the patient's dose so they receive the correct amount of the drug
    D) alert the pharmacist and have them prepare the compound

40. What is a characteristic of a paste?
    A) use of a dry ingredient
    B) an oily texture
    C) use of gelatin
    D) a thin texture

41. Which controlled substance is classified as a Schedule II drug?
    A) tranquilizers
    B) anabolic steroids
    C) opioids
    D) heroin

42. If a patient has a history of drug abuse, pharmacists may do all of the following EXCEPT:
    A) monitor controlled medications.
    B) put restrictions on controlled medications.

**C)** make sure the patient is complying with the directions.

**D)** tell a family member to monitor the patient's use of the medication.

**43.** Of the following medication pairs, which two are considered therapeutic substitutions for each other?

**A)** Lipitor and atorvastatin

**B)** Aciphex and pantoprazole

**C)** ciprofloxacin and amoxicillin

**D)** Plavix and metoprolol

**44.** iPledge is an FDA program that regulates the sale of:

**A)** isotretinoin.

**B)** tretinoin.

**C)** levotretinoin.

**D)** dextrotretinoin.

**45.** How many days' supply can be prescribed with one Schedule II prescription?

**A)** 7 days

**B)** 30 days

**C)** 60 days

**D)** 90 days

**46.** A 6-year-old boy is 126 cm tall and weighs 34 kg. The adult dosage of his prescribed medication is 400 mg. Using Clark's rule, the dosage for the boy will be:

**A)** 160 mg.

**B)** 200 mg.

**C)** 240 mg.

**D)** 300 mg.

**47.** The DEA requires all of the following to be on the prescription for a controlled substance EXCEPT the:

**A)** patient's date of birth.

**B)** patient's address.

**C)** prescriber's address.

**D)** prescriber's registration number.

**48.** At what temperature should the influenza vaccine be stored?

**A)** body temperature: 97.52 – 99.68°F (36.4 – 37.6°C)

**B)** room temperature: 60 – 86°F (15 – 30°C)

**C)** refrigerated: 36 – 46°F (2 – 8°C)

**D)** frozen: -4 – 14°F (-20 – 10°C)

**49.** Which of the following medications should be counted on a tray not used for other drugs?

**A)** methylphenidate

**B)** sertraline

**C)** penicillin

**D)** methylprednisolone

**50.** A patient's insurance will only fill generics manufactured by a single company. The patient fills omeprazole 40 mg with an NDC of 79534-1357-40. Which of the following NDCs would also be filled by this patient's insurance?

**A)** 52510-1357-40

**B)** 79534-9708-20

**C)** 95374-1357-30

**D)** 97453-8563-40

**51.** Which of the following pieces of equipment can a pharmacy technician use to measure the diluent required to reconstitute an oral liquid?

**A)** graduated cylinder

**B)** measuring cup

**C)** beaker

**D)** syringe

**52.** Which of the following questions from a patient can a pharmacy technician answer?

**A)** "Can I take Tylenol with this prescription?"

**B)** "How does this medication work in my body?"

**C)** "Does my insurance cover a ninety-day supply of this prescription?"

**D)** "What are the side effects of this prescription?"

**53.** The abbreviation *QID* means:

**A)** every day.

**B)** every other day.

**C)** four times daily.

**D)** three times daily.

54. Which of the following medications should NOT be stored on the common pharmacy shelf?

A) alprazolam

B) penicillin

C) chlorhexidine gluconate

D) lisdexamfetamine

55. If 1 L of a solution contains 5 g of a drug, how much of the drug would be present in 750 mL?

A) 1.5 g

B) 3.75 g

C) 2.75 g

D) 4 g

56. NDC numbers were implemented under which act?

A) Orphan Drug Act

B) FDA Modernization Act

C) Medicare Modernization Act

D) Drug Listing Act of 1972

57. Succinylcholine is primarily used for:

A) pain management.

B) chemotherapy.

C) anesthesia.

D) treatment of autoimmune disease.

58. Which of the following drugs is a high-alert medication?

A) metronidazole

B) potassium chloride injections

C) ketorolac

D) lisinopril

59. Dispensing the LASA drug clonidine in place of Klonopin may result in:

A) renal failure.

B) seizures.

C) hyperglycemia.

D) neuropathic pain.

60. Deteriorated drug errors occur when:

A) drugs that require specific laboratory values for dosing are not monitored properly.

B) drugs are administered whose potency and integrity have been compromised.

C) nurses fail to properly follow administration protocols.

D) the prescribed dose is not administered at the correct time.

61. How many mL of a solution containing 150 mcg/mL of medication would be needed if a patient requires a dose of 1 mg?

A) 5 mL

B) 3.33 mL

C) 6.67 mL

D) 7.5 mL

62. Tall Man lettering should be used for:

A) guanfacine and guaifenesin.

B) Depakote and diltiazem.

C) Avapro and Antivert.

D) Zovirax and zolpidem.

63. Which of the following written quantities correctly follows procedures for preventing medication errors?

A) 03 units

B) .7 units

C) 0.5 units

D) 100.00 units

64. What can workers do in a clean room?

A) garb

B) generate labels

C) prepare CSPs

D) wash hands

65. A patient with a prescription for rivaroxaban should be referred to the pharmacist if they are also purchasing:

A) aspirin.

B) acetaminophen.

C) diphenhydramine.

D) omeprazole.

66. A doctor prescribes methylprednisolone 10 mg tablets with the following directions:

6 tabs po qd for 2 days;

5 tabs po qd for 2 days;

4 tabs po qd for 2 days;

3 tabs po qd for 2 days;

2 tabs po qd for 2 days;
Then 1 tab qd for 5 days
How many tablets should be dispensed to fill this medication?

**A)** 25

**B)** 45

**C)** 50

**D)** 100

67. Which of the following medications is labeled with a boxed warning?

**A)** tamsulosin

**B)** lisinopril

**C)** allopurinol

**D)** pioglitazone

68. Which FDA recall level is used when there is a probability that the use of the product could cause an adverse event?

**A)** Class I

**B)** Class II

**C)** Class III

**D)** Class IV

69. Hydralazine is primarily prescribed to treat:

**A)** seizures.

**B)** depression.

**C)** hypertension.

**D)** diabetes.

70. If a prescription is presented for 180 g of a 7.5% cream and the pharmacy only stocks 10% and 2% strengths, how much of each strength would be needed to compound this order?

**A)** 123.75 g of the 10% and 56.25 g of the 2%

**B)** 140.25 g of the 10% and 39.75 g of the 2%

**C)** 125 g of the 10% and 55 g of the 2%

**D)** 110.88 g of the 10% and 69.12 g of the 2%

71. The drug class suffix *–pam* is used for:

**A)** benzodiazepines.

**B)** beta blockers.

**C)** antiviral medications.

**D)** SSRIs.

72. Which of the following entities is NOT covered by the guidelines described in HIPAA?

**A)** health care providers

**B)** health insurance plans

**C)** family members of the patient

**D)** health care workers

73. Pharmacy technicians write a large *X* on drug containers to show others that the:

**A)** drug is about to expire.

**B)** container has been opened.

**C)** medication is generic.

**D)** medication is brand name.

74. Which federal law required that prescriptions be written by a physician for certain medications before they can be dispensed to a patient?

**A)** Pure Food and Drug Act of 1906

**B)** Food, Drug, and Cosmetic Act of 1938

**C)** Durham-Humphrey Amendment of 1951

**D)** Comprehensive Drug Abuse Prevention and Control Act of 1970

75. Which two NDCs represent the same medication?

**A)** 23096-1980-92 and 23096-1890-92

**B)** 23096-1980-92 and 23096-1980-30

**C)** 23096-8940-92 and 23096-9840-92

**D)** 02934-9284-70 and 02934-9990-70

76. Which part of Medicare covers prescription drugs?

**A)** Medicare Part A

**B)** Medicare Part B

**C)** Medicare Part C

**D)** Medicare Part D

77. Which is NOT a law or requirement that was established under the Anabolic Steroids Control Act of 1990?

**A)** Anabolic steroids are not allowed to be prescribed in the United States.

**B)** Trainers and advisers cannot recommend anabolic steroid use to individuals.

**C)** Anabolic steroids must be classified as a Schedule III controlled substance.

**D)** Anabolic steroids are defined as a drug or hormonal substance that promotes muscle growth in a way similar to testosterone.

78. Which agency approves the use of investigational new drugs (INDs)?
   A) DEA
   B) CDC
   C) ASPCA
   D) FDA

79. What is a decentralized pharmacy?
   A) a system that alerts the nurse when the medication should be administered
   B) the center of pharmacy operations in a hospital or health care facility
   C) nursing unit med rooms that contain an automated dispensing machine
   D) the sterile room

80. How many tablets are in a tapering methylprednisolone dose pack that starts with 6 tablets on day 1?
   A) 14
   B) 21
   C) 31
   D) 64

81. How many times can a patient refill a Schedule III or IV prescription?
   A) zero times
   B) two times
   C) five times
   D) six times

82. Which of the following substances should be used to clean counting trays?
   A) isopropyl alcohol 90%
   B) isopropyl alcohol 70%
   C) witch hazel
   D) hydrogen peroxide

83. Which of the following suffixes is used for histamine-2 blockers?
   A) –olol
   B) –pril
   C) –tidine
   D) –artan

84. Which reference book is a resource on drug pricing?
   A) the *Orange Book*
   B) *Drug Facts and Comparisons*
   C) the *Red Book*
   D) Martindale's *The Complete Drug Reference*

85. A physician orders sodium chloride 20 mEq. The pharmacy only has sodium chloride 40 mEq/20 mL available. How much is needed to make the solution?
   A) 2 mL
   B) 6 mL
   C) 10 mL
   D) 12 mL

86. Which auxiliary label should be affixed to a prescription bottle of metronidazole?
   A) Shake well before use.
   B) Do not drink milk or eat dairy products.
   C) May cause drowsiness.
   D) Do not drink alcoholic beverages when taking this medication.

87. Child doses are calculated by the child's:
   A) weight.
   B) height.
   C) age.
   D) grade.

88. Which of the following is NOT required on a prescription label?
   A) patient's name
   B) directions for use
   C) insurance information
   D) patient's order number

89. A patient taking which of the following medications should be counseled to avoid alcohol?
   A) gabapentin
   B) potassium chloride
   C) naproxen
   D) ranitidine

**90.** Which of the following drugs does NOT treat osteoporosis?

**A)** raloxifene

**B)** ibandronate

**C)** zoledronic acid

**D)** methotrexate

# Answer Key

1. **A)** Salmeterol prevents asthma attacks and bronchospasms.

2. **A)** The patient will need 2 puffs BID (twice daily), so they will require 4 puffs a day. If the inhaler contains 60 doses, the supply will last 15 days (60 doses ÷ 4 doses/day = **15 days).**

3. **C)** If no day is given in the expiration date, the drug will expire on the last day of the listed month.

4. **D)** Enalapril is the generic equivalent of Vasotec.

5. **B)** DEA Form 106 is used for theft or loss.

6. **A)** Laminar flow hoods bring in and filter outside air to prevent contamination.

7. **D)** The drug's NDC number is not required.

8. **C)** Draw a tic-tac-toe grid and put the higher % strength in the top left square, the desired % strength in the middle square, and the lower % strength in the bottom left square. Then, subtract diagonally.

| 10 | | 3 |
|---|---|---|
| | 5 | |
| 2 | | 5 |

Add the numbers in the right column to find the number of parts: 3 + 5 = 8.

Divide the needed volume by the total parts: 250 mL ÷ 8 parts = 31.25 mL per part.

On the grid, multiply the numbers in the right column by the mL per part to find the final volume.

| 10 | | 3 × 31.25 = 93.75 mL |
|---|---|---|
| | 5 | |
| 2 | | 5 × 31.25 = 156.25 mL |

The 5% dextrose solution will be made from 93.75 mL of the 10% solution and 156.25 mL of the 2% solution.

9. **C)** Pantoprazole is the generic substitute for Protonix.

10. **A)** Extended-release medications should be swallowed whole, not chewed or crushed.

11. **D)** Set up a proportion with the number of capsules on top and the milligrams on the bottom. Five capsules of amoxicillin contain 2,500 mg of amoxicillin.

$$\frac{5\ \text{capsules}}{2,500\ \text{mg}} = \frac{x\ \text{capsules}}{50,000\ \text{mg}}$$

Cross-multiply and solve for $x$.

2,500$x$ = 250,000

$x$ = **100 capsules**

12. **A)** Meloxicam is an NSAID and should be taken with food or milk to minimize stomach irritation.

13. **A)** Tall Man lettering is used to differentiate among LASA drugs.

14. **D)** Warfarin is contraindicated during pregnancy because it affects fetal development and may lead to hemorrhage or spontaneous abortion.

15. **C)** Metronidazole is an antibiotic/antiprotozoal and is not a Schedule drug.

16. **A)** The letter *A* is used for providers who began practicing before 1985, and the second letter is the initial of the provider's last name. If Dr. Johnson began practicing in 1981, her DEA number would start with AJ.

17. **C)** Constipation is not a side effect of ciprofloxacin.

18. **B)** Noncontrolled prescriptions are good for 1 year from the date they are written.

19. **B)** Registered nurses do not have the authority to prescribe medications.

20. **D)** First set up a proportion with ounces on top and teaspoons on the bottom to determine how many teaspoons the patient must take to finish the 8 ounces.

    Use the fact that 1 fl. oz = 6 tsp.

    $$\frac{1\,fl.\,oz}{6\,tsp.} = \frac{8\,fl.\,oz}{x\,tsp.}$$

    $x$ = 48 teaspoons

    So 48 teaspoons are needed, and the patient must take 2 teaspoons every 4 hours, day and night; thus the patient needs 12 teaspoons a day.

    Therefore, the 8-ounce bottle (48 teaspoons) will last 4 days.

    24 hours ÷ every 4 hours = 6 times a day

    6 times a day × 2 teaspoons = 12 teaspoons a day

    48 teaspoons total ÷ 12 teaspoons = **4 days**

21. **A)** Doxycycline may cause tissue hyperpigmentation or tooth enamel defects in children with developing teeth and so is used with caution in children younger than 8 years. The pharmacist should counsel the customer on the potential side effects.

22. **A)** A counter balance is used for weighing non-sterile compound ingredients.

23. **B)** Edema is not a listed side effect of lisinopril.

24. **A)** Cough is a common side effect of ACE inhibitors.

25. **B)** The patient will take 1 tablet every 4 – 6 hours (up to 6 tablets a day) as needed for 10 days: 6 × 10 = **60 tablets.**

26. **B)** The two 250-mg capsules will be replaced with one 500-mg capsule. The patient will take 1 capsule twice a day for 10 days: 1 capsule × 2 capsules/day × 10 days = **20 capsules.**

27. **C)** Amoxicillin may be prescribed to patients under 18 years old. Paroxetine (Paxil) and escitalopram (Lexapro) are antidepressants, which may increase the risk of suicidal thinking and behaviors in children and adolescents. Aspirin may cause Reye syndrome in children with viral illnesses.

28. **C)** The abbreviation *T* means "tablet."

29. **C)** Orphan drugs are pharmaceuticals that are developed specifically for rare diseases.

30. **A)** Drinking grapefruit juice with lovastatin increases absorption and serum concentration of the drug.

31. **D)** The sig code for "repeat" is *rep, rept.*

32. **B)** The patient will take 1.5 tablets every day (40 mg × 1.5 = 60 mg). For a 30-day supply: 1.5 × 30 = **45 tablets**.

33. **D)** Ondansetron is used for nausea.

34. **B)** DAW-1 indicates that substitutions are not allowed by the prescriber. Doctors use this code when the brand medication is medically necessary, and substitution is not allowed.

35. **D)** The NDC number does not include the drug's expiration date.

36. **D)** Weight gain (not weight loss) is a common potential side effect of prednisone.

37. **A)** DEA numbers for manufacturers start with the letter *E.*

38. **D)** The quantity of the compounded medication would be on the medication label.

39. **A)** If a mistake is made during compounding, the technician should properly dispose of the incorrectly made compound and start the process again.

40. **A)** Pastes are thick, moist, and mixed with a dry ingredient.

41. **C)** Opioids are Schedule II drugs.

42. **D)** The pharmacist would be violating HIPAA by telling a family member to monitor the patient without the patient's permission.

43. **B)** Pantoprazole is a therapeutic substitution for Aciphex, a brand name of rabeprazole. Both medications are proton pump inhibitors.

44. **A)** iPledge is a Risk Evaluation and Mitigation Strategy for isotretinoin (Accutane).

45. **B)** A single Schedule II prescription can be filled for a 30-day supply.

46. **B)** Identify the formula and variables.

    Note that for Clark's rule, the child's weight needs to be in pounds, so you have to convert from kilograms (using dimensional analysis, a proportion may also be used).

    Recall that 1 kg ≈ 2.2 lb.

    $$\text{child's dose} = \frac{\text{weight of the child}}{150} \times \text{adult dose}$$

    $$\text{weight of the child} = 34 \text{ kg} \times \frac{2.2 \text{ lb}}{1 \text{ kg}} = 74.8 \text{ lb}$$

    adult dose = 400 mg

    Solve for child's dose.

    $$\text{child's dose} = \frac{74.8}{150} \times 400 \text{ mg} = \textbf{200 mg}$$

47. **A)** The DEA does not require the patient's date of birth to be on the prescription for a controlled substance.

48. **C)** The influenza vaccine is refrigerated at a temperature of 36 – 46°F (2 – 8°C).

49. **C)** Penicillins are a common allergen and should be counted on their own tray to avoid cross-contamination.

50. **B)** The first five digits of the NDC (79534) identify the manufacturer and would have to be the same for all this patient's generic prescriptions.

51. **A)** A graduated cylinder is used to reconstitute an oral liquid.

52. **C)** The pharmacy technician may answer questions about insurance but not about pharmacology (e.g., side effects, drug interactions).

53. **C)** The abbreviation *QID* means "four times daily."

54. **D)** Lisdexamfetamine (Vyvanse) is an amphetamine, a controlled substance, and should be stored in a locked cabinet.

55. **B)** Set up a proportion with milliliters on top and grams on the bottom. You need to convert 1 L into 1,000 mL so that the units match.

    1 L = 1,000 mL

    $$\frac{1,000 \text{ mL}}{5 \text{ g}} = \frac{750 \text{ mL}}{x \text{ g}}$$

    Cross-multiply and solve for *x*.

    $$1,000x = 750 \times 5$$

    *x* = **3.75 grams**

    This can also be solved using dimensional analysis, multiplying by conversion ratios to cancel out units until the needed units are found:

    $$750 \text{ mL} \times \frac{1 \text{ L}}{1,000 \text{ mL}} \times \frac{5 \text{ g}}{1 \text{ L}} = \textbf{3.75 g}$$

56. **D)** The Drug Listing Act of 1972 implemented NDC numbers.

57. **C)** Succinylcholine is a paralytic agent used in anesthesia.

58. **B)** Potassium chloride injections are considered high alert.

59. **B)** Clonazepam (Klonopin) is a benzodiazepine and antiseizure medication. Dispensing clonidine in its place may result in seizures.

**60.** **B)** Deteriorated drug errors are caused by using expired drugs or drugs whose chemical or physical potency and integrity have somehow been compromised.

**61.** **C)** Set up a proportion with milligrams (weight) on top and milliliters (volume) on the bottom.

You need to convert 150 mcg to 0.150 mg so the units will match.

150 mcg = 0.150 mg

$$\frac{0.15 \text{ mg}}{1 \text{ mL}} = \frac{1 \text{ mg}}{x \text{ mL}}$$

Cross-multiply and solve for x.

0.15x = 1 mg

**x = 6.67 mL**

This can also be solved using dimensional analysis, multiplying by conversion ratios to cancel out units until the needed units are found:

$$\frac{1 \text{ mL}}{150 \text{ mcg}} \times \frac{1,000 \text{ mcg}}{1 \text{ mg}} \times 1 \text{ mg} = \textbf{6.67 mL}$$

**62.** **A)** Guanfacine and guaifenesin are LASA drugs.

**63.** **C)** Leading zeroes should be used before decimal quantities, and trailing zeroes should not be used.

**64.** **C)** CSPs are prepared in a sterile room under a laminar airflow hood.

**65.** **A)** Aspirin is contraindicated with rivaroxaban because it increases the risk of bleeding.

**66.** **B)** The abbreviation *po* stands for "taken by mouth," and *qd* stands for "once a day" (for example, take 6 tablets orally once a day for 2 days).

Compute the number of tablets for each part of the prescription. Then, add up the total number of tablets for all the days.

6 tabs po qd for 2 days: 6 × 2 =1 2

5 tabs po qd for 2 days: 5 × 2 = 10

4 tabs po qd for 2 days: : 4 × 2 = 8

3 tabs po qd for 2 days: 3 × 2 = 6

2 tabs po qd for 2 days: 2 × 2 = 4

1 tab po qd for 5 days: 1 × 5 = 5

12 + 10 + 8 + 6 + 4 + 5 = **45**

**67.** **B)** Lisinopril has a boxed warning for potential fetal toxicity.

**68.** **A)** Recall level I is used when there is a probability that use of or exposure to the product could cause an adverse event or health consequences, or death.

**69.** **C)** Hydralazine is a vasodilator taken to manage hypertension.

**70.** **A)** Step 1: Draw a tic-tac-toe grid and put the higher % strength in the top left square, the desired % strength in the middle square, and the lower % strength in the bottom left square:

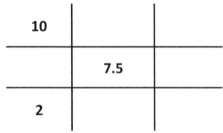

Step 2: Calculate the difference between the bottom left number and the middle number going up diagonally, and also the difference between the top left number and the middle number going down diagonally (ignore any negatives). Then add up those two numbers to get 8. This sum becomes the "parts" needed to work with.

| 10 | | 5.5 |
|----|----|-----|
| | 7.5 | |
| 2 | | 2.5 |

5.5 + 2.5 = 8 parts

Step 3: Now, divide the needed volume into the total parts: 180 g ÷ 8 parts, resulting in 22.5 g per part.

Step 4: On the grid, go back up to the parts and write the weight in g for each part.

| 10 | | 5.5 × 22.5 = 123.75g |
|----|----|-----|
| | 7.5 | |
| 2 | | 2.5 × 22.5 = 56.25 g |

So 5.5 parts of the 10% solution × 22.5 g = **123.75 g**, and 2.5 parts of the 2% solution × 22.5 g = **56.25 g.**

71. **A)** The drug class suffix –*pam* refers to benzodiazepines.

72. **C)** Family members are not HIPAA-covered entities.

73. **B)** An *X* is written on a container to mark that it has been opened.

74. **C)** The Durham-Humphrey Amendment of 1951 required that prescriptions be written by a physician for certain medications before they can be dispensed to a patient.

75. **B)** Two NDCs with the same four-digit product ID code (1980) represent the same medication.

76. **D)** Medicare Part D covers prescription drugs.

77. **A)** Anabolic steroids may still be prescribed in the United States.

78. **D)** The FDA (Food and Drug Administration) approves the use of INDs.

79. **C)** The nursing unit med rooms with automated dispensing machines are the decentralized pharmacy.

80. **B)** Tapering methylprednisolone dose packs have one less tablet each day: 6 + 5 + 4 + 3 + 2 + 1 = **21 tablets.**

81. **C)** A Schedule III or IV prescription can be refilled five times within six months from the original date.

82. **B)** Isopropyl alcohol 70% should be used to clean equipment such as counting trays and spatulas.

83. **C)** The suffix –*tidine* is used for histamine-2 blockers.

84. **C)** The *Red Book* is a resource on drug pricing.

85. **C)** Set up a proportion with mEq on top and milliliters on the bottom. Then, cross-multiply and solve for *x*.
$$\frac{40 \text{ mEq}}{20 \text{ mL}} = \frac{20 \text{ mEq}}{x \text{ mL}}$$
$$40x = 400$$
*x* = **10 mL**

86. **D)** Patients taking metronidazole should be counseled to avoid alcohol.

87. **A)** Child doses are calculated by weight and BSA.

88. **C)** It is not necessary to include insurance information on the prescription label.

89. **A)** Both gabapentin and alcohol are CNS depressants; combining them may result in lethargy, dizziness, or impaired mental abilities.

90. **D)** Methotrexate is an immunosuppressant.

Follow the link below to take your SECOND PTCB practice test:

**www.triviumtestprep.com/ptcb-online-resources**